pla
foreign

GW00691135

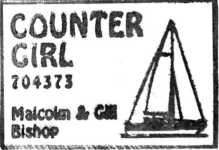

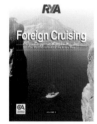

Information for yachts visiting the
Mediterranean and the Black Sea

A companion volume, *Foreign Cruising
vol 1 (C1)*, contains information regarding
countries on the Atlantic, including the
Canaries and Baltic seaboard.

Compiled from various sources

Revised by Clive Gardner

*With special help from Andrew Balint,
Jane Curtis, Sandy Duker, Roger Edgar,
Clive Garner, David Hide,
Jan Ledowchovsky, Mike Morris, Hasan
Kaçmaz and David Teall*

*Cover photograph:
A view from the top of the islet called
Stromboliccio towards the Stromboli with
its still active volcano. Bluegreen*

*Other photographs:
Premier Marinas and MDL.*

*Layout by Creativebyte
Printed by JPS Group*

Published jointly by

Cruising Association
CA House 1 Northey Street Limehouse Basin
London E14 8BT
Tel: 020 7537 2828
Fax: 020 7537 2266
Email: office@cruising.org.uk
Web: www.cruising.org.uk

The Royal Yachting Association
RYA House Ensign Way Hamble
Southampton SO31 4YA
Tel: 0845 345 0400
Fax: 0845 345 0329
Email: info@rya.org.uk
Web: www.rya.org.uk

CONTENTS

Should visitors find that regulations or practices differ from those described in these pages, information would be gratefully received and should be addressed to the Cruising Association or to the Royal Yachting Association.

The publishers wish to record their appreciation of the assistance received in the preparation of this book from many people, including embassies and tourist offices of the countries concerned, Cruising Association Honorary Local Representatives and numerous cruising yachtsmen who have written of their experiences.

Some regulations are more strictly applied than others. Where there is a difference of opinion, the official line has always been quoted. Local interpretation may be more or less rigid.

Whilst every effort has been made to ensure the accuracy of this publication, neither the compilers, the Cruising Association nor the Royal Yachting Association or any of their officers accept any responsibility for the results of any errors or omissions.

GENERAL INFORMATION

PURPOSE

This book has been written to help those planning to cruise to the Mediterranean and Black Sea areas. It details the regulations that apply to yachtsmen abroad and has other useful information to help them.

A companion volume, C1, covers the Atlantic Coast of Europe, The Baltic and Scandinavia.

Most of the information applies to boats owned by private individuals and taken abroad by them on a cruise of limited duration either lasting less than six months, or covering two or more seasons and involving laying-up in a foreign country before returning home.

More detailed advice will be needed by yachtsmen who plan:

- to base their boat outside the EU.
- to import their boat permanently into a country either inside or outside the EU.
- to cruise in a company-owned yacht.
- to offer their yacht for charter in a foreign country or use it for any other commercial purpose.

If you do so the rules regarding taxation, flag state registration and residency will vary considerably from those for vessels on short visits of up to six months. You are strongly advised to seek professional guidance from a lawyer or relevant authority of the country concerned. A list of addresses that can be used as starting points is given at the end of each chapter. Allow plenty of time!

Any such information printed within this guide is based on personal experiences and is intended purely to help people highlight potential areas for concern. It should not be considered to be the solution.

ORGANISATIONS

Yachtsmen planning to go foreign cruising should seriously consider becoming personal members of the Royal Yachting Association (RYA) and the Cruising Association (CA).

The RYA represents the views of the yachtsman as well as the other leisure boating sectors to the UK Government and, through affiliated organisations, to the EU and the international community. The RYA is the national association for sailing in the UK and is internationally recognised for the high standard it sets for both shore-based and practical training for leisure boat users.

The RYA has cruising and legal divisions, which combine to provide a one-stop centre for advice and help when planning to go foreign cruising. The RYA has comprehensive cruising FAQs (Frequently Asked Questions) on its website at www.rya.org.uk, which cover an increasing variety of cruising subjects from boat registration and VAT, to chartering and going foreign cruising. The RYA also offers sea safety information over the telephone, by email and via its website.

The CA has an English speaking honorary local representative for every area and many ports around the world who is available for help and advice when you urgently need a reliable marine engineer, a sailmaker or some important advice on laying-up. The CA library in London offers exceptional facilities for cruise planning. www.cruising-association.com

These two organisations have an important role in boating in the UK and in helping British sail and motor cruisers to cruise freely abroad and at home. Fly your ensign and burgee and remember the courtesy flag and your membership cards when you are sailing.

CUSTOMS

Pleasure craft arriving in and departing from the UK are subject to Customs regulations. These are described briefly below but full details can be obtained from Customs Notice 8, Sailing Your Pleasure Vessel To and From the UK. All HM Customs & Excise Notices are available from your local Customs office, as listed in the phone book, or from www.hmrc.gov.uk.

A vessel owned by a European Union resident is entitled to free movement throughout the EU, with no time limits, as long as the vessel has VAT paid status within the EU. However, it should be noted that some countries may enforce local regulations once a boat has been there for six months. It is also becoming usual to have to prove ownership, or the right to have control of the boat.

Vessels owned by non-EU residents and registered outside the EU are usually entitled to tax free Temporary Importation (TI) into the EU for up to 18 months. Longer periods may be granted for laying up or repair but Customs must be contacted in advance to arrange this concession.

Boats purchased VAT free in the EU by EU residents must leave the EU within two months at the date of delivery this is known as the Sailaway Scheme - Notices 8, 703/3, 703/2 refer.

Vessels registered in the Channel Islands cannot cruise under Temporary Importation rules unless the owner is a non-EU resident.

If you are planning to cruise to a non-EU country, there may be time limits for Temporary Importation of EU boats. Check with the relevant national tourist information office or embassy for details before you depart.

CUSTOMS PROCEDURES

Departure from any EU port direct to any other EU port

No action required.

Arrival in any EU port direct from any other EU port

No action is required unless you have something to declare such as firearms or non-EU nationals on board.

Some countries require reporting eg. Schengen Agreement.

Departure from any EU port direct to any non-EU port

Inform Customs. In UK, complete Form C1331 and post the top copy in a Customs Box before departure.

Arrival in any EU port direct from any non-EU port

Fly flag Q at 12 mile limit. Contact Customs - they will tell you what to do. Be prepared to prove the VAT status of the vessel. Tel: Yachtline 0845 723 1110.

Outside the EU

Practices vary; they are described in the corresponding chapters. If in doubt, skippers should:

- Fly flag Q on first entering territorial waters.
- If not boarded by Customs on arrival at their first port, present the Ship's Papers to the nearest Customs office.

Note: The Channel Islands, Gibraltar and Canary Islands are outside the VAT area of the EU.

European Economic Area (EEA)

This includes all countries of the EU and certain others such as Norway and Iceland. Countries belonging to the EEA are annotated below the country title in this book. Regulations between EU and EEA are changing fast. These changes will be announced as the RYA becomes aware of them in *RYA Magazine* or the RYA website: www.rya.org.uk.

IMMIGRATION AND HEALTH

It is the responsibility of the owner or skipper to:

- Report any cases of suspected infectious diseases.
- Ensure that non-EU passport holders obtain permission to land.

Customs officers often act for their country's immigration and health authorities but in some countries it may be necessary to visit several offices.

SCHENGEN AGREEMENT

A border free agreement known as the Schengen Agreement exists between many of the EU (not the new ones) countries, but not including the UK and Ireland.

NON EU RESIDENTS

Where applicable, details of procedures can be found in the relevant chapters.

The European Union has the following member states

Austria	Estonia	Hungary	Luxembourg	Slovakia
Belgium	Finland	Ireland	Malta	Slovenia
Cyprus	France	Italy	Netherlands	Spain
Czech Republic	Germany	Latvia	Poland	Sweden
Denmark	Greece	Lithuania	Portugal	UK

Temporary importation (TI)

Temporary Importation (TI) into these countries is only available to vessels:

    a) Registered outside the EU, and

    b) Owned by non-EU residents.

Boats subject to TI may not be lent to EU citizens or other non-entitled persons, chartered or sold during their time in the EU. If they are, they become subject to the normal rules for VAT.

Travel within the EU counts as if you are travelling within one country, because the EU is one VAT area. Customs officials may extend TI for bona fide reasons, eg:

- If the boat is laid up and unused.
- If the boat is undergoing refit or repair.
- If the owner leaves the EU.

Usually customs officials will only extend TI by short periods at a time, typically in six month sections. Application for an extension of TI should be made officially to the local customs authority and should be submitted well in advance.

There are a number of countries that are geographically situated within Europe, but which are outside the EU or the EU VAT area. A boat that has exceeded its TI limit may cruise in such countries without being subject to EU VAT rules. The following countries are close to the EU but not part of it. Note that some of them will have their own TI time limits.

The following maritime countries are outside the EU:

Albania	The Channel Islands	Iceland	Morocco
Algeria	Croatia	Israel	Norway
Bulgaria	Egypt	Lebanon	Romania
The Canary Islands	Georgia	Libya	Russia

Gibraltar is in the EU but outside the Customs zone.

In the past, Customs officials in France, particularly on the Atlantic coast, applied the TI rules very harshly. Vessels from outside the EU have been subjected to large fines and instant expulsion from the EU. We would strongly advise advance application for an extension of TI in this case.

Relief from VAT is available in certain cases when there has been a change of residence from outside the EU to inside it. There are more details on the RYA's website: check out the Cruising FAQs on www.rya.org.uk or from Revenue & Customs Notice 8 - on www.hmrc.gov.uk .

CERTIFICATES OF COMPETENCE

When cruising the coastal waters of most countries, it is usually sufficient to comply with the requirements of your own flag state. This is the country or state of registry of your boat. In the UK, skippers of boats used solely for private pleasure use are not required to hold any certificates of competence, but the levels of regulation for leisure boating vary widely. Some countries' officials are so used to demanding certificates of competence that they believe it is a legal requirement for everyone visiting their country and may delay boats where the skipper cannot prove competence to their satisfaction.

On inland, or internal, waters the situation is different. International Maritime Law states that the law of the coast state has precedence over that of the flag state. This means that the officials of the country you are cruising in can legally demand certificates of competence from the skippers of all boats on their internal waters. The various chapters in this book, under Documentation of Crew, will tell you if you need a certificate of competence for each country.

If you are going to cruise abroad it is wise to get a certificate of competence before you go. Ideally, the certificate should be issued by the Government of the skipper's country of residence.

For more information on certificates of competence see the Personal Papers section later in this chapter or the RYA's FAQ on the International Certificate of Competence (ICC) on www.rya.org.uk./cruising.

ANIMALS

The co-operation of every yachtsman is required to keep rabies out of those areas of Europe that are rabies free. The regulations on importation and quarantine of animals must be respected. Customs or the Coastguard should be notified of any yacht with animals aboard arriving in the UK.

Strict rules are imposed for transporting animals from one country to another, even within the EU. Therefore, vessels carrying animals must ensure that they familiarise themselves with the individual country's rules before they attempt entry.

The Pet Transport Scheme (PETS) does not allow animals to be imported or re-imported in the UK on private pleasure vessels. Only licensed carriers may bring in animals under the scheme on prescribed routes.

For more information about PETS call the helpline on 0870 241 1710 or consult the website: www.defra.gov.uk/animalh/quarantine/index.htm or email: pets.helpline@defra.gsi.gov.uk.

FLAGS

A yacht abroad must wear the national ensign of her country of registration. (British yachtsmen should be aware that the blue ensign may be misunderstood). It is illegal for a British vessel to fly as an ensign the EU flag, the Welsh Dragon or any flag other than the Red Ensign or special ensign. Other flags should be flown at the cross-trees. A permit from the authorised yacht club must be held by a person who wears any British ensign other than an undefaced Red Ensign and the appropriate burgee must be flown.

A courtesy flag of the country being visited should be flown from the starboard spreaders. It must be the top flag on the halyard. This courtesy flag is a small version of the maritime flag of the country being visited.

There is a FAQ on flag etiquette and the use of ensigns at www.rya.org.uk. Alternatively the RYA publishes a book called *Flag Etiquette & Visual Signals* (C4). You can buy it online at www.rya.org.uk/shop or by calling 0845 345 0372.

WEATHER FORECASTS

NAVTEX operates throughout the region giving weather forecasts and navigation warnings in text form, in English. NAVAREA 3 covers the area. NAVAREA 2 covers the Eastern Atlantic south of 48° N and including the Gibraltar Strait. Forecasts on VHF can be heard around most of the area. Texts of many of these various services can also be obtained on the Internet.

Broadcasting of Maritime Safety Information (MSI) is usually the responsibility of MRCCs but there are many other sources of weather forecasts. RYA G5 Weather Forecasts by David Houghton £4.75 contains details of most weather forecasts available in European waters. See, also, the CA weather site (www.franksingleton.clara.net)

The coast radio stations in the UK and in some other countries have closed. The Maritime Safety Information (MSI) services are the responsibility of the Coastguard within UK waters.

The RYA Book G22 VHF Radio is a useful reference to carry.

SHIP'S PAPERS

These typically comprise of:

- A registration document. This must be the original, not a photocopy.
- Evidence of marine insurance.
- The ship's radio licence.
- VAT receipt or exemption.

Each of these is explained in more detail below. In some countries it is compulsory to carry on board certain nautical publications or copies of local collision rules and regulations. This is particularly true when cruising on inland waters. Check the relevant country's chapter for details and see the section on Local Laws in this chapter.

REGISTRATION

RYA Cruising publishes Frequently Asked Questions (FAQs) about UK boat registration on the cruising pages of the RYA's website: www.rya.org.uk

There are two methods of registering a British yacht:

Full registration under Part 1 of the Merchant Shipping Act of 1995. This is open to all vessels whose owner is established in Britain. It is the only registration open to company owned yachts. It involves measurement, which can be organised through the RYA for craft less than 24m long. To arrange measurement, contact RYA Technical on 0845 345 0383 or email: technical@rya.org.uk.

Application forms for Part 1 Registration can be obtained from:

Registry of Shipping and Seamen,
PO Box 420,
Cardiff CF24 5XR
Tel: 029 2044 8800 or 8830/8841

Vessels registered on the Part 1 Register without a specific renewal date will need to renew their registration every five years. Part 1 Registration for Vessels with a build date prior to 1990 may have expired and should be renewed immediately.

If the year of build is unknown, renew as soon as possible as the registration may have expired.

The Small Ships Register (SSR) provides a simpler and cheaper form of registration for pleasure craft under 24m long and owned by UK, EU or Commonwealth citizens ordinarily resident in the UK. Registration lasts five years, or until a change of ownership, if earlier.

SSR registration can be completed and amended online at www.mcga.gov.uk (select The MCA, then Flagging into the UK).

Otherwise SSR information can be obtained from:

Registry of Shipping and Seamen,
PO Box 420,
Cardiff CF24 5XR
Tel: 029 2044 8800 or 8856/8857

The SSR does not record a vessel's tonnage and this has caused difficulties where dues are calculated on tonnage. The SSR does not have a port of registration. If required, use a convenient port which should be displayed on the boat.

British registered yachts based in France should not carry the name of a French port on the transom unless French registered and tax paid.

INSURANCE

Marine insurance is virtually compulsory; policy documents are often demanded in European countries. It is essential that territorial cruising limits are extended as necessary before the voyage is undertaken and then rigidly observed. Note that UK and Continent, Brest to Elbe may not necessarily include Ireland. Some countries require a minimum level of third party insurance and others, additional or instead of this, require a translation of all or part of the insurance document. Insurance is almost compulsory on all inland waterways.

Check the relevant country's chapter in this book or consult your insurance broker.

RADIO

A Ship Radio Licence is required for every yacht with R/T equipment installed. It can be obtained from:

Ofcom Radio Licensing Centre
Ship's Licences, PO Box 1495, Bristol BS99 3QS

Tel: 0870 243 4433 Fax: 0117 975 8911 Website: www.radiolicencecentre.co.uk

You can download licence application and renewal forms from www.radiolicenceforms.co.uk and apply or renew online. The ship's radio licence is not transferable between owners, and must be renewed if the vessel is sold.

It is now compulsory for most large commercial vessels to use the Global Maritime Distress & Safety system (GMDSS) and they are only compelled to keep watch on VHF Channel 16 'when practicable'. Since April 2001, it has not been possible to buy a radio unless it is compatible with Digital Selective Calling (DSC). The UK Coastguard is no longer required to keep a dedicated headset watch on Channel 16. A loudspeaker watch will be maintained for the foreseeable future with the provision to change to a headset watch if circumstances require.

Existing non-GMDSS radios fitted in private pleasure vessels are not affected by this legislation and can still be licensed and operated. It is only when buying a new boat or when fitting new equipment that the new regulations apply. All mariners (including recreational boaters) are urged to fit and use VHF DSC for distress and routine calling.

When operating radio equipment the appropriate operator's licence must be held. For VHF GMDSS equipment, this is the Short Range Certificate (SRC) and for MF/HF or INMARSAT equipment it is the Long Range Certificate (LRC). For non-GMDSS VHF, the old VHF-restricted Operator's Certificate is still acceptable as is the SRC. For details of how to get these qualifications check out the RYA website www.rya.org.uk or contact the RYA's Training Division by Email: training@rya.org.uk

It should be noted that the UK's coast radio stations have closed and those in some other countries are closing. Therefore the facility for making link calls no longer exists. Mobile phone, E-mail and satellite communications have taken the place of link calls.

Details of Inmarsat services and products can be obtained from:

INMARSAT Customer Service Centre
99 City Road, London EC1Y 1AX
Tel: 020 7728 1777   Fax: 020 7728 1142
E-mail: customer_care@inmarsat.com
http: www.inmarsat.com

For routine calls a VHF transmitter may only be used by a qualified operator or a person under the direct supervision of a qualified operator. Operators should note that on European inland waters VHF power is limited to 1W except on Ch 16. Ch 6 is for inter-ship business. Ch 77 is for inter-ship informal business. Increasingly all vessels are expected to be listening on the port operations channel. Some harbours require radio reporting.

The Rhine Countries

The Netherlands, France, Germany, Luxembourg and Switzerland, are known as the Rhine Countries where a new radio system known as ATIS is compulsory for boats based on the Rhine. Sea-going vessels are exempt from fitting the special radio equipment but are required to use 1W transmission power on all channels except Ch 16 and to use their ship's name and call sign each time they transmit. In addition, VHF Ch's 6, 8 and 72 may be used for personal messages. These requirements are in addition to the compulsory listening watch on local operational channels.

FIREARMS

A firearms certificate is required for a Verey pistol, Mark I mini-flares or the Nico signal flare system. A strong box must be provided if this equipment is present on board and they must be declared, with the original copy of the firearms certificate, when any border is crossed, this includes internal EU borders. The certificate is obtained from the police. Flares, other than those mentioned above, do not need firearms certificates. Hand guns, other than signalling apparatus, are banned in the UK.

PERSONAL PAPERS

These typically comprise:

- Passport (with appropriate visas as required).
- International Certificate of Competence.
- Maritime Radio Operators' Certificate of Competence and Authority to Operate.

In addition, some form of personal health insurance is advisable.

Each of these is considered in more detail below:

Passport

Every crew member must have a valid passport and any necessary visas. Passports are not required by UK citizens visiting the Republic of Ireland. Some countries require a minimum passport life e.g. in excess of six months before the expiry date, before permitting entry. Visa requirements for people arriving on a yacht are the same as arriving by more formal means such as a ferry, aeroplane or by car. Residency regulations should be investigated in advance if you are going to be in a country for more than 183 days in any 12 month period.

International Certificate of Competence (ICC)

Increasingly skippers of visiting craft are being asked for proof of their competence to operate the vessel they are driving and vessels can be delayed when no certifcate of competence is carried. Technically an RYA Certificate used on a UK flagged vessel should be entirely acceptable and some translations are available, which it is worthwhile carrying if you are intending to visit countries to which they are applicable. The International Certificate of Competence (ICC) is a much abused document, but in addition to being acceptable to countries which have adopted UN Resolution 40 under which the ICC is regulated, it does seem to do the trick with the local authorities in many countries including many EU member states which have not adopted the resolution. In fact Harbour authorities may well demand it in such countries (e.g. Spain and Greece).

The ICC also appears to be generally accepted by charter fleets irrespective of the nationality under which the charter yacht is registered, although this is outside the scope of the resolution. The RYA strongly recommends that you obtain and carry the ICC when cruising abroad. The ICC can be obtained from the RYA on completion of a test at an RYA affiliated club or an RYA Training Centre, or by proving successful completion of an acceptable RYA practical course. This should include taking the CEVNI test to allow the certificate to be endorsed for inland if you intend to venture inland at all. Further information on the ICC can be found at www.rya.org.uk under FAQs.

Maritime Radio Operators' Certificate of Competence and Authority to Operate

This must be held by someone on board (not necessarily the skipper) before marine radio equipment can be used for general communication. The VHF Restricted qualification is suitable for pre-GMDSS VHF equipment. If DSC equipment is to be used, either the Short Range Certificate (SRC) for DSC/VHF or the Long Range Certificate (LRC) for MF/HF GMDSS or INMARSAT equipment should be held. RYA Training can give details of courses and where to take them, see the RYA's website www.rya.org.uk or E-mail: training@rya.org.uk or telephone 0845 345 0384.

HEALTH INSURANCE

Health insurance policies should be examined to ensure that water-based activities are not excluded. In every case, the original document must be carried - not photocopies.

UK yachtsmen can obtain reciprocal emergency National Health cover in other EEA countries on production of Form E111. The form has be changed for 2005 and new style forms must be obtained from the post office as the old Form E111 is no longer valid. These new forms will only be valid until 31st December 2005 as during the course of 2005 the UK will be adopting the European Health Insurance Card. An associated book gives details of the cover available in EEA countries.

The Department of Health has a useful website: www.dh.gov.uk/PolicyAndGuidance/HealthAdviceForTravellers/fs/en with details of health risks around the world, where new Form E111 is available to download and further information on the EHIC is available.

VAT

The HM Customs & Excise website www.hmrc.gov.uk, lists all current notices. RYA Cruising publishes Frequently Asked Questions (FAQs) about VAT on the cruising pages of the RYA's website www.rya.org.uk.

When sailing between EU countries it is important that evidence of VAT paid status of the vessel is carried. This appears to be particularly important in Spain, Portugal, Greece and France. This evidence could be any of the following options:

- The original VAT receipt received at the time of purchase.
- The VAT receipt for subsequent payment on import or at the outset of the Single Market.
- The Customs acceptance of relief from VAT, i.e. on change of residence from outside the EU. UK Customs Notice 8 (available on their website or from the Customs offices) has the details.
- Proof that the vessel was taken into use prior to 1st January 1985 (1987 for Austrian, Finnish and Swedish vessels) and was lying in the EU on 1st January 1993 (1 January 1995 for Austrian, Finnish and Swedish vessels). Similarly, for most recent EU member states: Cyprus, Czech Republic, Estonia, Hungary, Latvia, Lithuania, Malta, Poland, Slovakia and Slovenia the vessel must have been in use prior to 1st May 1996 and in the EU on 30th April 2004.
- Acceptance by your national customs authority that the vessel is of tax paid status.

In the absence of any of the above, a Bill of Sale showing that the boat changed hands between two private individuals in the UK will normally suffice. This is not the conclusive proof that VAT has been paid on the vessel, it advises the foreign customs official that the tax status of the vessel is in the business of UK Customs. It is still advisable to check the required documentation with the relevant authorities or their UK Embassy in advance of your voyage.

Note that if the vessel was in Temporary Importation on 1st January 1993, the customs authority of that country must issue the documentation.

ROAD VEHICLE PAPERS

The papers required when taking a boat abroad on a trailer typically comprise:

- The vehicle registration document.
- International Driving Licence (outside the EU).
- Evidence of insurance for boat and trailer. The insurance Green Card is required in most countries and should always be carried. Some countries also require separate cover for a trailer. Your insurer can advise.
- Customs Carnet (in some countries only). The chapter for each country indicates whether a Carnet or Customs Bond is required. This guarantees to the host country that the tourist will not sell his boat or engine tax-free while in the country. It can be obtained from the AA or RAC.
- Some form of breakdown and recovery insurance, to cover the trailer as well as the car, is prudent.
- In most European countries, the overall length of vehicle and trailer may not exceed 18m, width 2.5m. Exceptions are indicated in the relevant chapters. The AA or RAC will provide detailed information and documentation for specific countries.

The RYA produces an information booklet called *Trailing and Roof Racking* which is useful for those wishing to tow boats. Contact RYA Legal (see page 89 for details).

LOCAL LAWS

Laws vary from country to country - as does the treatment of offenders. A hobby which involves the use of binoculars and cameras can be misunderstood, especially near military installations.

On the inland waterways of mainland Europe the Code Europeen des Voies de Navigation Interieure (CEVNI) rules replace the COLREGs. These require different standards of lights, both in position and brightness. Dispensation is given to vessels arriving from the sea, but if you are based on the inland waters you should comply with CEVNI. If in doubt, do not travel at night. An English summary of CEVNI is available from the RYA - G17 The RYA European Waterways Regulations (The CEVNI Rules Explained) £6.85 +75p P&P, either online or by calling direct see page 89 for RYA contact details).

Some countries require copies of local regulations to be carried on board. If using inland waterways: Holland requires the carriage of the Inland Waterways Police Regulations (BPR) found in Volume 1 of the ANWB Almanac for Holland; France requires the carriage of the Inland Water Signals and Regulations (CEVNI) available from RYA as above.

ANTI DRUGS ADVICE

All yachtsmen are asked to be alert to the use of vessels for the transportation of illegal drugs. If you notice unusual activity, at sea or in remote coastal areas, do not attempt to involve yourself, but report the facts as soon as possible to the local Customs authorities. If there is a language barrier you may prefer to contact the British Consulate. Information can be given anonymously in the strictest confidence and should not be broadcast on VHF. To avoid problems, crew members on serious medication should carry a letter from their doctor. This should state what the drug is and for what complaint. You can play your part in the fight against drugs wherever you are. Drug offences are now punished by massive fines, confiscation of the yacht and long imprisonment. Do not carry parcels for other people. Anti-drugs Alliance confidential hotline 0800 59 5000.

CONSULAR ASSISTANCE

British Consulates exist to help British citizens abroad to help themselves. On arrival in a foreign country it is sensible to note the address and telephone number of the local British Embassy, High Commission or Consulate (see the local telephone directory or ask at the tourist information office). A Consul's resources and the help he can give are limited.

If necessary he/she can:

- Issue an emergency passport.
- Advise on how to transfer funds.
- Advise on procedures in case of death or accident.
- Contact British nationals who have been arrested.
- Tell you about organisations who can trace missing persons.
- Cash a small sterling cheque supported by a banker's card.
- Possibly, as a last resort, make a loan towards repatriation to the UK.

He/She cannot:

- Get you out of prison.
- Get you better treatment in hospital or prison.
- Give legal advice.
- Investigate a crime.
- Get you a work permit.
- Pay your bills.

It is sensible to ensure that, in case of disaster, every crew member has sufficient money to buy a ticket home from the furthest point likely to be reached on the cruise.

NAVIGATION

There are no Loran C transmissions in the Mediterranean or Black Sea. There have been recent developments and it is planned to use it as an integrity check for GALILEO - the emergent EUROPEAN Satnav system.

The datum point for GPS is WGS 84. Many national hydrographers, including the UK Hydrographic Office are currently running programmes to update charts to WGS 84. Charts referenced to WGS 84 will be boldly overprinted with this information so it is wise to check which datum your charts are based on. If they are different to the satellite datum, most GPS sets can be programmed to the datum on the chart or, if not, it is possible to calculate corrections for datum differences. Contact the UKHO for further details on 01823 337900. www.ukho.gov.uk

DUTY FREE STORES

Yachts planning to voyage beyond the Elbe (actually the north bank of the R.Eider) or Brest are permitted to embark stores duty free in the UK. It is necessary to provide a suitable locker into which the stores can be sealed by a Customs officer until the yacht has left UK waters. The value of this concession to a yacht making a coastal voyage is limited because most countries allow only the normal tourist allowance to be withdrawn from the sealed store whilst the yacht is in their territorial waters. It is necessary to make a written application to Customs who may make a charge for their services. Customs point out that this is not a statutory entitlement, but rather a concession that they allow.

It is permissible to import unlimited quantities of alcohol, perfume and cigarettes bought tax paid in one EU country into another EU country as long as they are for personal use. Keep the receipt to prove tax status.

Beware of importing excess duty free goods from the Channel Islands into the EU.

At present, duty free red diesel is available for yachts in the UK, Ireland, Belgium and Finland and fuel may be carried in the main tank to other EU countries. However, loose containers of red diesel may not be acceptable. It is advisable to keep all receipts to prove its origin.

PUBLICATIONS

In each of the following chapters there is a list of useful publications for that country. In addition, the Cruising Association's *Cruising Information Series* includes publications covering the French (and Belgian) Inland Waterways, the Western Mediterranean, the Adriatic, Greece and Turkey, each providing an introduction to cruising in those waters at greater length than this book can include. The CA also publishes annual updates to the principal Mediterranean pilot books, compiled from reports by members.

A variety of useful publications, including the European (CEVNI) Regulations book, pilot books and leisure craft charts are available to buy from the RYA either online from the RYA Shop at www.rya.org.uk/shop or from RYA Despatch. (see page 84).

For more information and a list of other suppliers see page 89.

MOBILE PHONES

If planning to use a mobile phone, ensure that international roaming and voice mail, etc have been set-up prior to departure from the UK.

International calling from and to mobiles on a UK account can be very expensive. If you are staying for some time in another country, it may be worth opening a local account and using their simcard.

The Europe-wide emergency number for mobile phones is 112.

CHEQUES

Eurocheques are no longer accepted.

SOLAS V

The International Maritime Organisation (IMO) is the UN specialised agency responsible for maritime safety and preventing pollution from ships. IMO is responsible for the International Convention of the Safety of Life at Sea, which is better known as SOLAS. SOLAS is one of the oldest Conventions of its kind and the first version was adopted in 1914 after the sinking of the Titanic with the loss of more than 1500 lives. The Convention is not a static piece of international law and is often revised and refined.

Since 1st July 2002, the following SOLAS regulations have been applied to all vessels owned by British nationals and of less than 150 gross tonnage:

Regulation 19.2.1.7 - If practicable, vessels must have a radar reflector or other means, to enable detection by ships navigating by radar at both 9 and 3GHz.

Regulation 29 - An illustrated table describing the life-saving signals shall be readily available to the person on watch. Ships or persons in distress shall use the signals when communicating with life-saving stations, maritime rescue units and aircraft engaged in SAR ops.

Regulation 31 - Skippers must communicate information about navigational dangers to the Coastguard using any means at their disposal. The Coastguard must promulgate this information. Such messages are free of charge to ships.

Regulation 32 - This regulation details the kinds of navigational dangers that should be communicated and has examples of danger messages.

Regulation 33 - Distress messages - obligations and procedures. Skippers are obliged to respond to distress messages from any source. The master of a ship in distress or the SAR authorities can requisition ships.

Regulation 34 - Safe navigation and avoidance of dangerous situations:

- Voyage planning on all vessels which go to sea.
- Master to ensure plan is drawn up.
- Details of factors to take into account.
- Master's discretion in decision-making not to be compromised (ie by owner or charterer of the ship - particularly with regard to large, commercial ships).

Regulation 35 - Distress signals only to be used for the proper purpose and must not be misused.

More information about these regulations are available from the RYA's website: www.rya.org.uk - see the FAQs.

FRANCE AND CORSICA
(Member of the European Union)

CRUISING

The French Mediterranean coast stretches for 300M between the Spanish and Italian frontiers. In the west is the Languedoc-Roussillon region and the Camargue. There are numerous large new marinas.

The Côte Bleu

The Côte Bleu runs from the Rhône to Toulon; there are small fishing harbours, marinas and the major port of Marseilles.

Côte d'Azur and Riviera

Further east is the very fashionable area of the Côte d'Azur and Riviera. There are many marinas, the facilities are excellent but they can be expensive and crowded. Cruising tends to be from one marina to another.

Corsica

Corsica is one of the most beautiful islands in the Mediterranean with numerous anchorages and small harbours, as well as marinas at Porto Vecchio, Bonifacio and Calvi. Some anchorages can be crowded at the height of the season but it is possible to cruise in comfort at other times.

Harbours and marinas

Along the French coast there are 60 good sized and many smaller ports and marinas. All are to a high standard.

Navigational aids

Buoyage and lights are good both on the mainland and Corsica.

Inland waterways

Main rivers and canals between the English Channel and the Mediterranean

The minimum lock dimensions for most of the waterways are:

Length: 38.5m

Draught: 1.8m

Beam: 5.0m

Height: 3.4m

These are known as the Freycinet dimensions, named after a Minister of Public Works who did much to upgrade the network circa 1880. A barge close to these dimensions is known as a peniche.

Exceptions

The Seine as far as Paris is navigable by boats drawing up to 3m with a maximum height of 6m.

On the Canal du Nivernais the maximum height is 2.7m, the maximum draught is officially 1.2m, but there has been silting and it is not recommended for boats drawing more than 1m.

On the Canal de Bourgogne the height of the tunnel at Pouilly-en-Auxois is only 3.1m, draught is 1.4m, and bulging lock sides currently reduce the maximum beam to 4.5m.

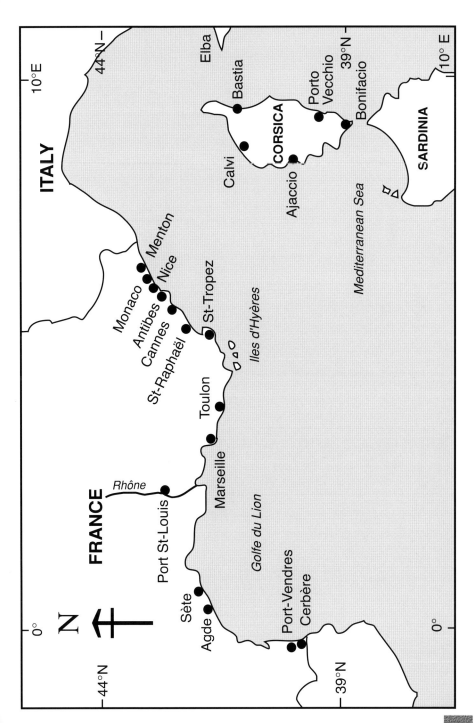

Canal du Midi between the Atlantic and the Mediterranean

Length: 30.0m

Draught: 1.5m In late or dry summers the depth may be reduced to 1.4m or less.

Beam: 5.5m

Height: 3.0m to the centre of the bridge arches. (Height at sides may be as low as 2m.)

Further information on the Rhône can be obtained from:

Service de la Navigation
2 Rue de la Quarantine 69321
Lyon Cedex Tel: 04 72 56 59 00
Fax: 04 72 56 59 01

These figures are a guide only. It should be recognised that water levels can vary with traffic, and especially in the south, with the amount of water extracted (usually overnight) for irrigation.

The carriage of masts across France while vessels navigate the inland waters can be arranged by:

Navy Service
Av. 1ère Div. Francaise Libre
13230 Port St Louis
Tel: 04 42 11 00 55   Fax: 04 42 48 45 06

Chantier Naval de la Baie de Seine
136 Quai Frissard 76600 Le Harve
Tel: 02 35 25 30 51   Fax: 02 35 24 44 18

The cost is likely to be about £500 incl taxes.

In principle, it is forbidden to discharge toilets into canals and rivers, but pump out stations are few and far between, and discreet overboard discharging is tolerated. However, this situation is beginning to change, usually as a result of local rather than national initiatives, and particularly in regions where the pleasure traffic predominates over commercial.

The introduction of a maximum 35 hour working week in France in 2002 has led to a general reduction in the operating hours of locks (and lifting bridges), especially on the Freycinet gauge and smaller waterways, and on summer weekdays, operation is usually from about 09.00 to 19.00, often with a one hour lunchtime closure. On Sundays it may be an hour or so less. The winter hours are shorter, usually restricted to daylight, and some waterways with little or no commercial traffic, are closed from November to March inclusive. With the reduction in working hours, local variations have replaced what were formerly fairly standard hours. Check locally or refer to the VNF website.

A list of scheduled *chromages* or lock and bridge closures can be obtained from late March or early April each year from the French Government Tourist Office, and is also published on the VNF website.

A licence or vignette is required on all the waterways managed by the VNF. This can be obtained at one of the VNF offices, which include Rouen, Le Havre, Calais and Dunkirk, or by post from the VNF headquarters in Bethune. For a personal application, note that most offices are closed at weekends, and not all are open full office hours during the week, so check by phone first. Addresses are available from the French Government Tourist Office, or the VNF website. Licences can be purchased for 16 consecutive days, 30 not necessarily consecutive days, or a full year. The tariffs, which are based on the product of the length and beam of the craft, are modest compared with their British equivalents.

Licences should be displayed on starboard side, forward.

On a few waterways, the use of old motor tyres as fenders is forbidden, because of the risk of their causing lock gates or paddles to jam should they become detached. On others, they must be attached to the vessel by two lines. In fact they are a useful addition to normal fenders, since they sink and can protect the hull below the waterline when mooring to sloping banks etc.

ENTRY

If a vessel is registered in an EU country it is not necessary to undertake any clearance, however vessels may still be checked by French Customs.

Ports of entry

A list of ports of entry is not published; all major ports have Customs and Immigration offices.

Entry by road

EU Customs regulations apply.

Generally speaking, provided that you comply with the regulations for towing in the UK, you will have complied sufficiently with French trailing law.

If the overall length of vehicle and trailer (including the boat) exceeds 18m, or if the width is greater than 2.5m, you must seek police permission to travel as a large load.

Customs

EU regulations apply.

Fly a yellow 'Q' flag only if you have something to declare. Yachts may be boarded by French Customs patrols up to 20km from the coast or in harbour. Customs may visit vessels inland as well as at ports of entry, and as well as inspecting ship's and crew's papers, may also check that untaxed (red) diesel is not being used. If there is red diesel in the ship's tanks, you must be able to show that it was purchased outside France, preferably by producing receipts and a record of all recent fuel purchases.

French police now have the power to forbid, temporarily or permanently, a foreign helmsman from driving a craft in French waters, but they have emphasised that this would only be enforced in cases of severe infringement of the French circulation rules.

Documentation

of vessel

Ship's registration papers, the original, not a photocopy, must be on board at all times.

The only craft exempt from this rule are those small enough to be classified as engin de plage (beach toy), for a definition see Appendix A.

The original of the yacht insurance policy must be carried on board.

of crew

EU regulations apply.

Passports

No Schengen declaration need be made.

Certificates of Competence

Note: The RYA is authorised by the UK Government to issue the ICC.

Coastal waters - British flagged boats

There is no requirement for skippers to hold a Certificate of Competence, or for British flagged boats to carry particular prescribed equipment when cruising the French coast.

Coastal waters - French flagged boats

Helmsmen of sailing vessels in French coastal waters do not need a licence, even if the boat is equipped with an auxiliary engine. A motorsailer may be counted as a motor boat, if its engines exceed the size laid down, by a special formula the French use to determine categories.

The helmsmen of French flagged motorboats will need either a Carte de Mer (for craft powered by engines between 6hp and 50hp, operating in daylight hours within five miles of a harbour), or a Permis de Mer (for craft outside these limits).

These French certificates are not available outside France, but a foreigner carrying a certificate of competence issued on behalf of their own government may drive a French flagged leisure motorcraft covered by that certificate.

French inland waters

Skippers of vessels navigating French inland waters need to hold a valid certificate of competence. The only exception is craft less than 5m in length and not capable of more than 20kph.

Category C licence - coches de plaisance. For those driving vessels less than 24 metres in length.

The 'new' ICC (issued since May 1999 and subject to UN Resolution number 40) is accepted. Holders of ICCs issued prior to May 1999, are restricted to using vessels up to 15m in length. ICCs must be valid for inland waters, which means the CEVNI test must have been passed.

For vessels between 24m and 39m in length, a category PP licence (Peniche de Plaisance), or a national certificate recognised by the French Government on a basis of reciprocity, is required. For vessels of any greater lengths only a commercial master's certificate will be valid.

In all cases, a copy of the CEVNI rules must be carried on board. The RYA G17 'European Waterways Regulations' is acceptable. It is available from the RYA's website, priced £6.85 plus postage. Alternatively, the code Vagnon Fluvial, in French, is well illustrated and offers a painless way of learning a little navigational French.

Only persons aged over 16 may helm on French inland waters. In general terms the French inland waters begin at the first obstacle to navigation for sea-going ships. On major rivers the start of inland waters is defined as -

Garonne, Pont de Pierre in Bordeaux.

Dordogne, Pont de Pierre in Libourne.

Loire, Pont Handandine or Pont de Pirmil.

Rhone, Pont de Trinquetaille in Arles.

Seine, Pont Jeanne d'Arc in Rouen.

On smaller rivers the mouth, excluding the coastal town, is taken as the limit of inland water.

Dutiable stores/animals

EU regulations apply.

Temporary Importation

EU regulations apply.

On the Atlantic coast of France, non-EU visitors have been fined for spending more than 6 months in any 12 in the EU. Non-EU visitors should not visit France if they been in the EU for more than 6 months in the last 12 without first checking with French Customs. Once a non-French EU citizen has been in France continuously for 6 months, a boat tax, known as a Passport, is payable.

OTHER INFORMATION

The unit of currency is the Euro.

Tel. code from the UK: 00 33

Tel. code to the UK: 00 44

To contact a yacht from ashore in France the number to call is 0801 011 021. The caller must state the name of the vessel, its call-sign and the name of the person required, also details of the area in which the yacht is cruising and the type of radio on board.

Clean mooring zones have been established in 10 selected bays between La Ciotat and Menton. Yachts are encouraged not to discharge sewage and this will eventually become mandatory.

Persons resident in France or other EU countries for more than six months may attract residential status and be subject to local taxes and regulations.

Fuel and stores

There is little problem in obtaining provisions of all kinds from shops, supermarkets and markets. Camping Gaz, diesel and water are readily available in all ports, but payment on unmanned, automatic fuel pumps may only be possible with French credit cards. Canal side refuelling points are infrequent, except where there is significant pleasure hire boat traffic.

Red diesel is only available for use in generators or in central heating systems and must not be used for the boat's engines. However red diesel in the tanks when a vessel arrives in France may be used. It is wise to retain a receipt to prove purchase outside France. Red diesel imported in cans is liable to duty.

French Butagas is easily obtainable and requires only a special regulator (d'Etendeur) for use with Calor appliances.

Many of the marinas have good repair and laying-up facilities. Spares can generally be obtained or shipped from the UK without too much difficulty.

Chartering

A list of charter companies operating in France is available from the French Government Tourist Office.

Inland waters charter companies operating on the French inland waters have a special dispensation from the Government which means that their clients may not have to hold ICCs. This dispensation is only valid when operating in certain restricted areas on charter boats. It expires at the end of the charter period and does not negate the need for skippers of privately owned boats to hold an ICC.

Weather forecasts

Every harbour office (Capitainerie) will display the forecast from Météo France on a daily basis. On the Côte d'Azur Monaco Radio now broadcast continuously in French and English as follows:

VHF Channel 23 Menton to St Raphael

VHF Channel 24 Corsica

VHF Channel 25 St Raphael to Port Carmague

Other stations broadcast forecasts as follows:

Néoules	Ch79	at 0815, 1233 & 1903
Agde	Ch79	at 0715,1245 & 1915
Planier	Ch80	at 0733, 1303 & 1933
Mont Coudon	Ch80	at 0745, 1315 & 1945
Pic de l'Ours	Ch80	at 0803, 1333 & 2003

Telephone forecasts are available on 36 68 08 + the two relevant departmental digits. Principal stations are:

Marseilles	1906kHz; 2649 - 3792kHz
Monaco	8728kHz.

Full details of French forecasts are available in a pamphlet issued by Météo France, available at most French Harbours and Marinas or direct from:

Météo France. 1 Quai Branly, 75340 Codex 07 Tel: 0145 56 71 71 and online at www.meteo.fr/meteonet/decouvr/guides/marine/marl.htm.

A subscription service for faxed synoptic charts and area forecasts can be arranged by writing to Météo France at this address.

Publications

Admiralty Sailing Directions Vols I & II

South France Pilot (several volumes) Brandon (Imray)

Mediterranean France and Corsica - A Sea Guide. Heikell (Imray)

Votre Livre de Bord - Meditérranée (Interval Editions), 3 Rue Fortia, 13001 Marseille

Tel: 04 91 54 38 97 Fax: 04 91 33 35 67)

CEVNI rules - G17 RYA European Waterways Regulations (The CEVNI Rules Explained) £6.85

Useful addresses

French Consulate General
21 Cromwell Road, London SW7 2DQ.
Tel: 020 7838 2000 or 020 7073 1200

French Government Tourist Office
178 Piccadilly, London W1V 0AL
Tel: 0906 824 4123 (premium rates) Fax: 020 7493 6594
www.francetourism.com

Touring Club de France
178 Piccadilly, London W1V 0AL

Touring Club de France
Champs Elysées, 75008 Paris
Tel: 01 42 65 90 70

Fédération Française de Voile (FFV)
50 Rue Kléber, Paris.
Tel: 01 47 04 90 12

Centre de Renseignements Douane
8 Rue de la Tour des Dames, 5009 Paris
Tel: 01 55 04 65 30

Ministères des Transports
Direction Général des Transports Intérieurs,
Direction des Transport Terrestres (sous Direction des Voies Navigables),
244-246 Boulevard Saint Germain, 5007, Paris.

Service Hydrographique et Océanographique de la Marine (SHOM)
BP 426, 29275 Brest
Tel: 02 98 03 09 17

VNF - Direction of Development
175 Rue Ludovic Boutleux
62408 Bethune Cedex
Tel: 0321 63 24 54
www.vnf.fr (French only)

General information on inland waterways can be requested from:
VNF - Inland Waterways Navigation Authority
175 Rue Ludovic Boutleux
62408 Bethune Cedex
Tel: 0321 63 24 54
www.vnf.fr (French only)

Appendix A

Definition of a Beach Toy (Engin de Plage)

The rule requiring registration of boats is relaxed for Beach Toys. These craft are not permitted to go more than 300m offshore.

They are defined as follows:

Rigid craft:

1. Rigid single-handed sailing craft and canoes:
    Beam less than 1.15m and product of length x beam x depth less than $1.5m^3$.
2. Other rigid craft (sail or motor):
    Beam less than 1.2m and product of length x beam x depth less than $2.0m^3$.

Dinghy sailors will find that the dividing line falls somewhere between a Laser (which requires registration) and a Topper (which is exempt).

Inflatable craft:

1. Motorised inflatables:
    Length less than 2.75m and beam less than 1.2m and air volume less than 350 litres
2. Sailing inflatables:
    Length less than 3.7m and sail area less than $7m^2$

Other craft exempt from registration:

1. Windsurfers (Sailboards)
2. Aquabikes (Jet-skis)

SPAIN
(Member of the European Union)

CRUISING

The Mediterranean coast of Spain has several major traditional cities, Barcelona, Valencia and Alicante, together with a considerable number of tourist developments and marinas. The Balearic Islands form a delightful cruising ground. Some small fishing ports are available to visiting pleasure craft. Care should be taken with the security of a yacht left unattended in the larger ports.

Spanish yacht clubs tend to be very exclusive and expect high standards of dress and behaviour from their members. Visitors are likely to be welcome only if they respect this attitude.

The Cabrera Archipelago, south of Mallorca, is a National Park and a permit (free) is required. Application should be made three weeks before required via local marinas or:

Tel: (971) 465507 (Palma de Mallorca).

Fax: (971) 465700.

Harbours and marinas

The Spanish Tourist Office publish detailed maps listing marina and harbour facilities, instalaciones nauticas, covering the regions of Andalucia, Balearics, Catalonia. A number of marinas provide lifting-out facilities.

ENTRY

Ports of Entry

There are no specified ports of entry, but if arriving from a non-EU country the first entry must be made at a port large enough to include a Customs office.

Entry by road

EU Customs regulations apply.

Customs

EU regulations apply.

Documentation

of vessel

• Ship's registration certificate, ship's radio licence and evidence of marine insurance cover in Spanish should be carried as should proof of VAT status.

At least the registration certificate, insurance certificate and all passports will have to be shown at nearly every port along the coast.

of crew

• A certificate of competence is required for the person handling the vessel. It is therefore advisable to have an ICC.

Spanish harbour charges

Harbour dues - Tarifa T-5 and T-0

Tarifa T-5, known in some places as G-5, is a harbour tax charged by the Province and applicable to all pleasure vessels although few skippers appear to be aware of its existence. When applied to long stay boats, the tax is levied twice a year, 1st March and 1st September, and is payable in advance. If arrangements are made to pay by standing order there can be a discount. The daily rate in Valenciana province is calculated as 0.0304 x L (metres) x B (metres), ie about €1 for a

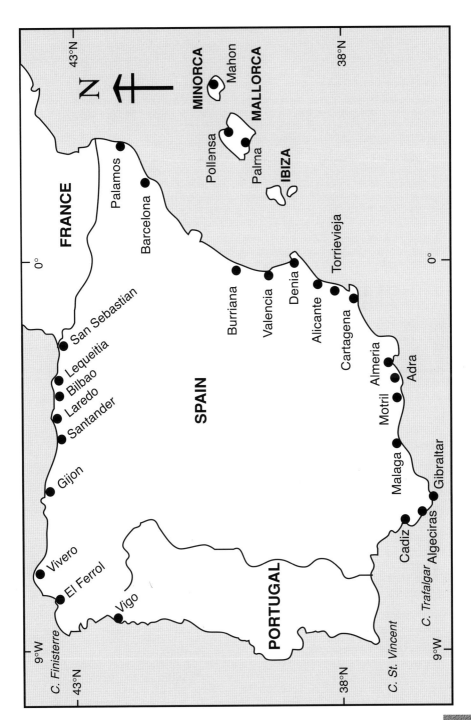

FRANCE

SPAIN

PORTUGAL

MINORCA

Mahon

MALLORCA

Pollensa

Palma

IBIZA

43°N

38°N

0°

9°W

Palamos

Barcelona

San Sebastian

Lequeitia

Bilbao

Laredo

Santander

Gijon

Vivero

El Ferrol

Vigo

Burriana

Valencia

Denia

Torrievieja

Alicante

Cartagena

Almeria

Adra

Motril

Malaga

Gibraltar

Algeciras

Cadiz

C. Finisterre

C. St. Vincent

C. Trafalgar

43°N

38°N

0°

9°W

N

10 m vessel. In some cases, the fee for long stay boats is payable direct to the Province. For short stay boats the tax may not be collected or it may be built into the marina charges.

Light dues, known in some places as Tarifa T-0, seem to apply to those renting or owning a berth for a period exceeding 6 months. Like T-5 it is payable in advance and, if paid promptly, can attract a discount. If boats in transit are charged then it will be through the marina fee.

Failure to pay either tax can result in boats being impounded and then charged the full rather than a discounted rate. Charging of both taxes seems to vary greatly from place to place. Anyone leaving a boat in a port is advised to clarify with the marina or harbourmaster regarding liability to any dues not included in the marina fees.

Wealth Tax

Spain levies a Wealth Tax (patrimonio) on residents and non residents alike. Your wealth is calculated by totalling your assets and deducting your liabilities and includes boats. There is a general allowance for residents against Wealth Tax of approx. €110,000 per person, property attracts a further €15,000 approx. There is no allowance for non-residents. As a rough guide a vessel worth €170,000 would attract a tax rate of 0.2% or €340.

Local interpretations may well differ and the situation may change. A non-Spanish national keeping a boat in Spain is strongly advised to make enquiries, of other owners, marina managements and, if in any doubt whatsoever, a Gestor (tax accountant).

OTHER INFORMATION

The unit of currency is the Euro.

Tel. code from the UK: 00 34

Tel. code to the UK: 00 44

STD calls may be made to the UK from public call boxes which have instructions in English.

Non-Spanish nationals living in Spain for more than six months in any one year are required to re-register their vessels on the Spanish register, thereby attracting a 12% registration tax and a requirement to comply with all Spanish licensing and equipment carriage regulations. They may also be liable for local taxes and compliance with other local regulations.

Chartering

There are numerous charter companies which operate in Spain and the Balearics and advertise in the major yachting magazines.

Insurance

There are minimum requirements for Third Party cover and for material damage. A Spanish language certificate to this effect must be carried on board. Get up-to-date advice from your insurer.

Fuel and Stores

Diesel is available at most ports and Camping Gaz is universally available. It is not easy to get other sorts of gas cylinders filled. Paraffin is difficult to obtain but 'lamp oil' is available in some large supermarkets and DIY stores. There are good repair facilities in many of the marinas and local workshops. Spares and electronic equipment are available in the larger marinas. There are excellent markets for fish, fruit and vegetables. Water is readily available and is normally potable. Wine, beer and local spirits are cheap and plentiful. A permiso aduarnero form from Customs will enable stores to be imported duty free.

Weather forecasts

Sea area and coastal weather forecasts are broadcast in English and Spanish, on marine VHF, almost everywhere from Huelva to the French border, including the Balearic Islands. There are also coastal forecasts in Spanish only. NAVTEX stations at Tarifa (G), Valencia (W) and Toulon (T) broadcast relevant weather forecasts. Radio Monaco, 3AC broadcasts the text of the Toulon

INMARSAT-C forecasts covering most of the western Mediterranean in English and French. For schedules, see ALRS Vol 3(1), RYA G5 and www.inm.es/web/sup/ciencia/divulga/infesp/metmar/zoncos.html

Forecasts for an area up to 5 NM from Gibraltar are broadcast on FM by BFBS and Gibraltar Broadcasting Corporation. Most marinas have weather forecasts posted on notice boards and there are many other sources of weather forecasts. See the CA weather site. (www.franksingleton.clara.net)

Holding tanks and heads

Spanish registered yachts and motor boats, regardless of age, are required to have holding tanks. The following rules regarding discharge of sewage apply to all vessels -

- In port waters, protected zones, rivers, bays, etc, discharge is not permitted, even with treatment.
- Up to 4 miles from shore, discharge with treatment is permitted, however there must be no solids and no discoloration of the water.
- From 4 miles to 12 miles, discharge is permitted if crumbled and disinfected. When discharging, the speed of the vessel must be more than 4 knots.
- More that 12 miles offshore, discharge is permitted in any condition. When discharging, the speed of the vessel must be more than 4 knots.

Publications

British Admiralty charts are excellent for use in Spanish waters and the information is now largely obtained from Spanish charts. Spanish charts, fully updated, are published by Instituto Hydrografico de la Marina at Cadiz and are obtainable there, or at any Libreria Nautica. Electronic charts also available.

Admiralty Sailing Directions
Mediterranean Pilot Vol 1
Mediterranean Spain, RCC Pilotage Foundation (Imray) (two volumes)
Islas Baleares, RCC Pilotage Foundation (Imray)
Imray M series charts, M1, M2 & M3.
Marina Guide – Mediterranean (Vetus).
In Spanish - Derroteros - which contains excellent pictures of the coast.
Instalaciones Nauticas (Spanish Tourist Office).

Useful Addresses

Spanish Embassy
24 Belgrave Square, London SW1X 8SB
Tel: 020 7235 5555

Spanish Consulate
23 Manchester Square, London W1M 5AP
Tel: 020 7589 8989

Spanish National Tourist Office
22-23 Manchester Square, London W1M 5AP
Tel: 020 7486 8077 Fax: 020 7486 8034
www.spaintour.com (In English)

Spanish Chamber of Commerce
5 Cavendish Square, London W1M 9HA
Tel: 020 7637 9061

Direccion General de la Marina Mercante
Ruiz de Alarconi, 28014 Madrid

Real Club Nautico de Barcelona
Tiglado 9, Barcelona

Federacion Espanola de Vela
Juan Vigon 23, Madrid 3

Real Automovil Club de Espana
General Sanjurjo 10, Madrid 3

Salon Nautico International, Avda
Reina Maria Christina, Palacio 1, Barcelona
Liga Naval Espanola
Silva 6, Madrid

Camper & Nicholsons (Spain) SA
Club de Mar, Palma de Mallorca, Spain

RHINE-DANUBE LINK

GENERAL INFORMATION

With the opening of the Main-Donau Canal in September 1992, a major new route from Western Europe to the Black Sea and the Eastern Mediterranean was available for yachts drawing under 1.8m and with masts unstepped. In 1999, the NATO bombing of Serbia destroyed many of the Danube bridges, especially at Novi Sad, thus rendering the river unnavigable. By end of 2002 the route had been cleared of broken bridges and unexploded bombs. Most of the bridges have now been or are being rebuilt, but in the centre of Novi Sad there remains a temporary pontoon bridge, which is only opened to river traffic a few times a week.

A replacement bridge is currently being built (the Sloboda Bridge) and once this is in use, the pontoon bridge will be dismantled. This is scheduled for early summer 2005.

For yachts not capable of cruising at more than 6-7 knots the route leads from England via the French canals to Strasbourg, down the Rhine to Frankfurt, up the Main, and through the Main-Donau canal to join the Danube at Kelheim. From Kelheim the rest of the journey is downstream on the Danube until the Black Sea is reached via the canal link near Constanta in Romania.

Vessels with enough power to cruise at 10 knots can also consider reaching the Main by travelling upstream on the Rhine, either from the Mosel or all the way from Holland. The 1.8m draft restriction mentioned above is imposed only by the French canals, and 2.5m is available by taking the route through Holland. The Main is completely canalised and currents are negligible. The Danube, although canalised, is quite fast-flowing, especially when it is in flood. Vessels without a great deal of engine power should avoid such times, even for a downstream passage, as harbour entry manoeuvres can be dangerous when the current is strong. Similarly, upstream passages are likely to be impracticable at any time for slow-moving vessels.

The Rhine Regulations require the skipper and active crew to be below stringent blood alcohol levels when under way – recently reduced to about half the permissible level for car drivers. Enforcement is strict, especially in Germany.

The Danube is an international waterway, and the formalities required are few. It is necessary, however, for each crew member to obtain a transit visa for the passage through the Serbian section of the river. This can be done, without having to produce an invitation, either in London or in Budapest. Holders of EU passports do not require a Romanian visa.

Documentation

of vessel

- Ship's registration papers, ship's radio licence and insurance certificate should be carried. Rhine Regulations must be carried when on the Rhine, CEVNI regulations in France and BPR (Inland Waterways Police Regulations) in Holland.

- Vessels longer than 20m will probably have to comply completely with local vessel requirements. These are likely to be full commercial specifications and are contained on the Règlement de visite. All vessels must comply with the Règlement de Police.

of crew

- Valid passports and International Certificates of Competence (ICC) with the CEVNI rules endorsement are necessary.
- Vessels of more than 15m must carry a Rhine pilot when navigating the Rhine and a Danube pilot in Austria. A Rhine sportsboat patent (licence) is available for vessels of 15m - 20m but this demands 16 recent voyages on the part of the river for which the licence is issued and is therefore effectively only available to locals. No such licence exists in Austria.

Publications

Maps/quides covering the route from Holland to the Black Sea are available from two German publishers, DSV-Verlag and Edition Maritim, both of Hamburg.

The Danube – A River Guide. Rod Heikell. (Imray)

G17 RYA European Waterways Regulations (The CEVNI Rules Explained) £6.85 – available from the RYA

Useful addresses

Hungarian Embassy Consulate & Visa Section
London SW1X 8BY
Tel: 020 7235 2664
Visa Information 0900 117 1204 (premium rate)

Romanian Consulate
4 Palace Green, London W8 4QD
Visa information 0900 188 0828 (premium rate)
Consular section 020 7937 9667

Commission Centrale pour la Navigation du Rhin
2 Place de la République, 67082 Strasbourg Cedex
Tel:+03 88 52 20 10   Fax: +03 88 32 10 72

GIBRALTAR
(Member of the European Union but outside VAT area)

CRUISING

The number of yachts calling at Gibraltar increases year by year and the facilities available to yachtsmen are also increasing. The two original marinas, Sheppards and Marina Bay, have both increased the available moorings, and there is a new marina development, Queensway Quay, inside the harbour. It is also possible for vessels to anchor to the north of the airport runway, but this entails a long trip in the dinghy to reach the shops.

Gibraltar has much to offer the visitor in terms of historic interest, fortifications, the rock and natural caves. The Government of Gibraltar is trying hard to promote tourism, consequently entry formalities are fairly relaxed.

ENTRY

by sea

On arrival skippers should report to the Customs reception berth next to the Shell refuelling station on the starboard side of the approach to the two older marinas. Queensway Quay has its own clearance facility.

by road

The frontier with Spain is fully open, although sporadic problems continue. Short stay trailed craft should have no difficulty in entering Gibraltar provided that the regulations for bringing a boat into Spain have been met (see chapter on Spain).

Customs

All items to be brought in duty free must be declared.

1. Upon arrival you are required to supply a crew list in triplicate.
2. To obtain clearance to go ashore travel documents, e.g. passports and, if appropriate, visas are required.
3. Any crew member or passenger intending to reside ashore during the time the vessel is in port must report to the Immigration Control Office, Waterport (0930 - 1300 Mon - Thurs. 1530 - 1700 Fri).
4. If any person on board has employment in Gibraltar, it must be reported to the Immigration Control Office.
5. Before leaving, report time and date of departure to the Immigration Control Office.
6. Immigration control must be advised of any guest residing aboard.

Although this may sound rather bureaucratic, CA members passing through recently found the atmosphere quite relaxed compared to Spain.

Documentation

of vessel

*   Registration document, insurance certificate. If the skipper of the yacht is not the owner then he should have a document, in English and Spanish, authorising the use of the vessel.

of crew

*   Passports

Dutiable Stores

Duty free liquor and tobacco may be readily obtained from any wine and spirit merchant on leaving Gibraltar.

Temporary Importation

There is no duty payable on the importation of a yacht into Gibraltar if the owner is not classified as a resident. A resident, for these purposes, is defined as a person who has stayed, or will stay, in Gibraltar for an average of six months or more per year over a period of three years previous to, or subsequent to, the date of importation. However, this rule is interpreted by the Customs authorities to mean that after a continuous stay of eighteen months, or aggregated in a period of less than three years, duty becomes payable. This period may be extended at the discretion of the Collector of Customs. The rate of duty is 12% of the yacht's value at the time of importation.

Gibraltar is part of the EU but outside the EU VAT area. Items being sent out of Gibraltar for repair must first be cleared with Customs and upon return be clearly marked 'spares in transit'.

OTHER INFORMATION

Tel. code from the UK: 00 350

Tel. code to the UK: 00 44

Although Gibraltar has its own sterling notes, British notes can be obtained from the banks. Both are legal tender.

Gibraltar has its own airport with direct flights on most days to the UK and Tangier.

Chartering

Two charter companies operate in Gibraltar; Enterprise Sailing (01491 572497) and International Charter Centre (01703 455069). Both advertise in British yachting magazines.

Fuel and stores

Petrol and diesel can be obtained at reduced duty rates at the Shell refuelling berth which is adjacent to the Customs reception berth.

Queensway Quay will arrange fuel delivery to the marina cheaper than that available from Shell or Esso.

There is a plentiful supply of English goods at Tesco and Safeway, close to the marinas. Excellent and comprehensive yacht repair services are available.

Weather Forecasts

Available in English on 1458kHz at 0645, 0730, 1230, and 2359 local time. Also regular VHF broadcasts (monitor Ch16). See also the section on weather forecasts in Spain, page 26.

Publications

Admiralty Mediterranean Sea Pilot Vol 1

North African Pilot (Imray).

Yacht Scene - Sailors' Guide - D M Sloma

Useful addresses

Gibraltar Information Bureau
National Tourist Office, 179 The Strand, London WC2R 3DT
Tel: 020 7836 0777

Royal Gibraltar Yacht Club
Queensway
Tel: 350 78897

Sheppard's Marina
Waterport
Tel: 350 77183/75148   Fax: 350 42535

Gibraltar Tourist Office
Cathedral Square
Tel: 350 79336
www.gibraltar.gi

Principal Immigration Officer
Waterport, Marina Bay Complex Ltd, PO Box 373
Tel: 350 73300   Fax: 350 78373
Queensway Quay Marina
PO Box 19, Ragged Staff Wharf
Tel: 350 44700   Fax: 350 44699

Gibraltar Chart Agency Ltd
Watergardens, Block 5, Unit 11a
Tel/Fax: 350 76293

ITALY
(Member of the European Union)

CRUISING

Italian Riviera

The Italian Riviera from the French border to Tuscany is a beautiful coast with much to offer, including numerous well-equipped marinas. This popular area is crowded in the summer months.

Tuscan coast

The Tuscan coast and archipelago offer marinas, harbours and anchorages which will also be crowded in summer, especially July and August when visitors' berths are at a premium.

Tyrrhenian seaboard

The northern part of the Tyrrhenian seaboard of Italy is crowded because of the proximity to Rome, and local yachts leave little space for the visitor. South of the Bay of Naples the coast is less busy.

Sardinia

Sardinia is a beautiful cruising ground, uncrowded except in the north east from mid-July to end of August. The western coast of Sardinia is rather exposed with limited safe shelter and should be navigated with due attention to the weather.

Sicily

The northern part of Sicily is an interesting cruising area and gives access to the various islands in the southern part of the Tyrrhenian Sea. The southern coast of Sicily is not well known as a cruising area but contains some of the finest archaeological sites outside Greece and Turkey.

East coast and 'toe' to the 'heel'

The toe to the heel of Italy is not popular for cruising but is useful for passage making to Greece and Croatia.

The east coast of Italy is not an attractive area for visiting yachts.

Venice to Trieste

The north coast from Venice to Trieste has many marinas where both Italian and foreign yachts are kept.

Italian lakes

Special rules apply on the Italian lakes. They are displayed in various languages at the lakeside. Documents must be carried on board.

Harbours and marinas

There are many marinas, fishing ports and anchorages and the Italian Waters Pilot is the best source of information in English. Many marinas in the popular areas are very crowded in the season, then it is best to phone or e-mail to reserve a berth in advance. Italian marinas can be very expensive, especially in the high season (July and August). Not all accept credit cards.

Navigational aids

There is good buoyage and lights as well as numerous radio beacons.

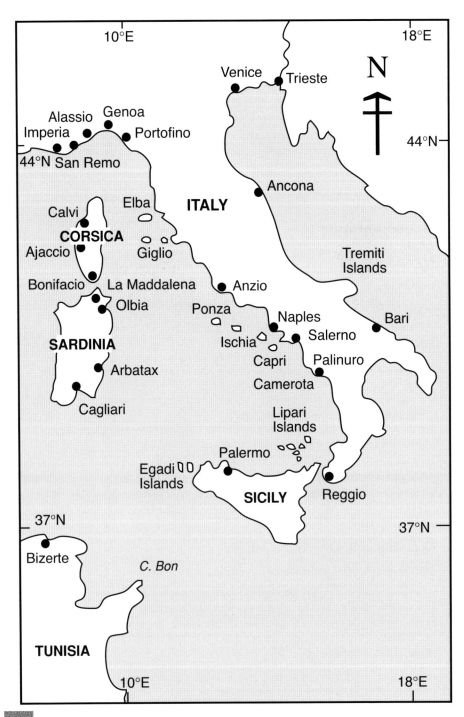

ENTRY

Ports of entry

There are no specific ports of entry; any major port will have customs and immigration facilities.

Entry by road

No customs papers are needed for boats with or without engines or when brought by car and trailer and having the same number plate. Boats must be inspected by a Port Authority before entering the water on some lakes. Boats with engines require insurance with the third party clause translated into Italian.

Customs

EU regulations apply.

Temporary importation

EU regulations apply.

Documentation

of vessel

- Ship's registration papers.

- A certificate of insurance with an Italian translation; this may not always be asked for but is nonetheless essential. The regulation concerned states that a visiting foreign yacht must have 'a Certificate of Insurance for third party liabilities issued by an Insurance Company having reciprocal arrangements with a recognised Italian Insurance Company'. It is therefore advisable to check with one's insurance company that this recognition exists, when asking them to supply the translation.

- Third party insurance complying with the regulation may be obtained in Italy quite cheaply through an insurance broker - the document is then, of course, in Italian.

- Proof of VAT status should be carried.

- A crew list is useful. It should read: surname, forename, date and place of birth, function on board, passport number and nationality.

- Foreign registered yachts are regularly checked for valid documentation by the Guardia di Finanza, especially if they are used for chartering.

of crew

- EU regulations apply.

- Foreigners carrying a certificate of competence from their own country may navigate the craft for which they are qualified. It is advisable to carry the International Certificate of Competence (ICC), particularly on motor cruisers.

OTHER INFORMATION

Tel. code from the UK: 00 39

Tel. code to the UK: 00 44

For making international calls the British Telecom International Card (or its US equivalents) often provides the cheapest call method. Peak rates are Monday to Friday, 0800 to 1300.

The mobile telephone network is extensive and heavily used. Check with your UK operator their preferred Italian network to be used for international roaming. For longer term stays use of an Italian SIM card will prove to be a cheaper solution than using a UK SIM card.

The unit of currency is the Euro. Banking hours are from 0830 to 1300 and for one hour in the afternoon - generally 1500 to 1600. Often there are security doors and all handbags and other packages must be left outside in lockers.

Travellers' cheques in Euros, together with a UK passport, are accepted by most banks and are preferred for getting cash (US Dollar or UK Sterling Travellers cheques are also accepted). Alternatively most banks have ATMs which will accept the main UK debit cards and credit cards for cash withdrawal.

Chartering

The Italian Tourist Board should be able to supply a list of yacht charterers.

Fuel and stores

Yacht repairs of all kinds are available in the major centres. Many marinas have lifting facilities. In smaller harbours help is usually available although it may be from a garage rather than a marine engineer.

Provisions are easily obtained from supermarkets and general stores, though some newer marinas are out of town with shopping facilities that are only open during the high season period. Diesel and water are available in most marinas and harbours, but in some islands the water must be paid for separately. Camping Gaz is readily available in shopping areas and chandlers. Credit cards are now usually accepted for fuel purchases for yachts.

Recreational Craft Directive

Italian law links boat design categories to an authorised area in accordance with the EU Directive.

Flags

The maritime flag of Italy consists of a defaced ensign, which is the correct courtesy ensign to fly from the starboard yardarm. It should be noted that most reference books show, and most UK chandlers sell, the national flag not the maritime flag.

Weather forecasts

The national radio station (Radio Uno) broadcasts forecasts in Italian for the whole of the Mediterranean at around 0640, 1530 and 2235 on 658kHz, 1035kHz and 1575kHz. The forecasts are read slowly and are easy to follow.

Monaco radio on SSB on 4363kHz, 8728kHz and VHF Ch 20 & 23 at 0903, 1403 and 1915 local, gives good forecasts in French followed by English.

There is a (nearly) continuous weather broadcast on VHF Ch 68 that is available in most areas. There are forecasts at 0135, 0735, 1335 and 1935 UTC, on various marine VHF channels, preceded by a call on Ch 16.

There are NAVTEX weather broadcasts from Rome [R], Cagliari [T] Augusta [V] and Trieste [U].

The Ch 68 and NAVTEX forecasts cover a 12 hour period with a 12 hour outlook followed by an outlook for the next 48 hours in 12 hour time slots. The other VHF forecasts are only for the first 24 hours. All these forecasts are identical and are for sea areas. The system is highly, but poorly, automated and there will be occasions when forecasts are incomplete. There is virtually no attempt to include any coastal effects.

For the Bonifacio Strait, the French CROSS forecast for Corsica is very useful.

Some marinas have forecasts of a more localised nature than the Italian broadcasts.

Toulon NAVTEX usually gives a better and more useful forecast service than the Italian.

Details of other useful forecasts can be found on the CA weather site. (www.franksingleton.clara.net)

Publications

It is wise to obtain BA Charts of the areas one intends to visit before leaving the UK as this avoids possible linguistic and conventional sign problems, but Italian charts are easily readable and up to date. In many areas the Italian large scale charts provide more extensive coverage than do the Admiralty charts, e.g. off the smaller Tuscan, Flegree and Pontine islands. They can be obtained in large ports (e.g. Genoa and Naples) from the Italian Naval Authorities and from many marina and harbour yacht chandlers or dive shops.

BA Charts and Pilot Books cover the whole area. Most yacht chandlers sell large scale plastic covered yachting charts but these are rather expensive.

The Tyrrhenian Sea, Denham (John Murray). Now out of print.

Admiralty Sailing Directions, Mediterranean Pilots Vols. 1, 2 and 3. (NP45, NP46 and NP47.)

Admiralty List of Radio Signals, Small Craft Edition, NP289 (Note: This is the only English language book which provides telephone numbers for most ports and marinas)

Italian Waters Pilot, 5th Edition. Heikell (Imray) 1998. (Currently being revised)

Adriatic Pilot, 3rd Edition, Trevor & Diana Thompson (Imray) 2000.

North Africa Pilot, 2nd Edition, Hans van Rijn & Graham Hutt (RCC Pilotage Foundation) 2000. This gives details of Italian islands off the western and southern coasts of Sicily.

Imray also publish via their internet site yearly updates for all the above three Pilots. These provide details of changes and corrections since the Pilot was published.

Pagine Azzurre, Il Portolano dei Mari d'Italia, published annually in Italian and is available from most chandlers in Italy. It gives detailed harbour plans and other useful information, e.g. the high season charges and port and marina telephone numbers. This can be of value even to those with very limited Italian.

Votre Livre de Bord, Méditerranée. (Bloc Marine) published annually in French, covers Sardinia and the west Italian coast from the French border to Livorno and is available from most yacht chandlers and marinas in France. It gives detailed harbour plans and other information which can be of value even to those with very limited French.

There are numerous other Italian and French cruising guides generally covering only the western side of Italy.

Vade-Marino for National Tourism in Italy (Italian State Tourist Board).

The normal tourist guides, such as the Rough Guide, can also be an invaluable source of information, e.g. for transport details, sights to see and places to visit, etc.

Useful addresses

Italian Consulate General
38 Eaton Place, London SW1
Tel: 020 7235 9371

Ente Nationale Italiano Turismo - Italian State Tourist Board
1 Princes Street, London W1B 2AY
Tel: 020 7408 1254   Fax: 020 7399 3567   E-mail: italy@italiantouristboard.co.uk
www.italiantourism.com

Federazione Italiana Vela
Via Brigata, Bisagno 2, Genoa, Italy
Tel: 00 39 010 56 50 83

Federazione Italiana Motonautica
Via Cappuccio, 19 Milano.

Federazione Italiana Sci Nautico (water skiing)
Viale Rimembranze di Greco, 1 Milano.

Federazione Italiana Canottaggio (rowing)
Viale Tiziano, 70 Roma.

GREECE
(Member of the European Union)

CRUISING

Greece offers the yachtsman a great variety of picturesque places to visit.

Aegean or Ionian Seas

Aegean or Ionian Seas, remote or cosmopolitan islands, rocky or pine fringed beaches, quiet anchorages or sophisticated marinas. Everywhere are splendid reminders of the classical past from the site of the first naval engagement at Salamis to the cruising grounds of Ulysses. Supplies and provisions are readily available except on the more remote islands. Water can be in short supply on some islands.

The Ionian Sea

The Ionian Sea, extending from Corfu to Zakynthos (about 140 miles) together with the Gulfs of Patras and Corinth (about 100 miles).

Saronic and Argolic Gulfs

The Saronic and Argolic Gulfs, extending from the eastern end of the Corinth Canal to the south eastern coast of the Peloponnese (about 120 miles).

Cyclades

The Cyclades, the large group of 21 main islands in the central Aegean (about 120 miles W/E and 120 miles N/S).

Evia and Northern Sporades

Evia and the Northern Sporades, which include Skiathos and Skopelos.

Northern Aegean

The Northern Aegean, including Limnos, Lesvos, Khios and Samos (about 150 miles North to South).

Dodecanese

The Dodecanese, the Twelve Islands (actually 14) on the eastern side of the Aegean, stretching from Patmos in the north to Rhodes in the south (about 100 miles N/S).

Crete, and Southern Peloponnese

Crete, and the Southern Peloponnese, including Kithera (about 250 miles from Zakynthos to Heraklion).

Harbours and marinas

There are hundreds of harbours and anchorages from which to choose. Most harbours are small fishing ports and not suitable for leaving a yacht unattended. There is a growing number of modern, fully-equipped marinas in Greece. The principal ones are:

Gouvia (Corfu)

Levkas (Ionian)

Vounaki (Palairos, Ionian)

Patras

Kalamata (Peloponnese)

Zea (Athens area)

Vougliameni (Athens area)

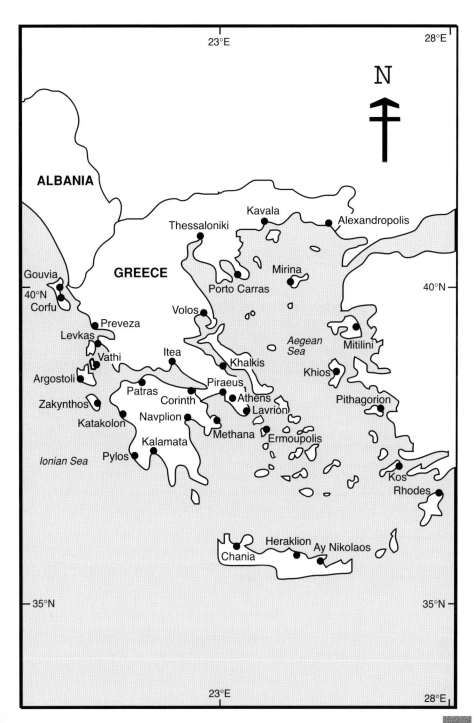

Kalamaki (aka Alimos, Athens area)

Glifada (Athens area)

Faliron (aka Flisvos, Athens area)

Methana (Saronic)

Olympic (Lavrion)

Thessaloniki (aka Aretsou)

Porto Sani (Thessaloniki)

Porto Carras (Khalkidiki)

Porto Gouves (Heraklion, Crete)

Mandraki (Rhodes)

It may be worth calling ahead to reserve a berth, especially in July and August.

It is still possible to find creeks and coves with good shelter, room to swing, fine scenery and not another yacht or house in sight. In harbour it is customary to berth bow or stern to quay wherever there is room and to avoid the berth used by the inter-island ferries. Blue and yellow diagonal stripes painted on a portion of the quay indicate the refuelling point for yachts. This berth must be left free if you are not refuelling.

Harbour Dues

Charges are made in all marinas and some, but by no means all, harbours. Harbour dues are collected by the Port Police on the basis of a complicated calculation related to LOA, not always consistently applied, and by no means always collected. The amounts invoiced are not substantial, with a charge of around €6 being average for an 11 metre boat.

All yachts (including EU and Greek flagged) must obtain a "DEKPA" - "Private Pleasure Maritime Traffic Document". For this there is a flat charge of €30.00. This is a 6-page A3 booklet. This must be presented to and stamped by the port authority on entry to and exit from each port visited, and is valid for a year or two until all 50 boxes are full.

For non-EU vessels the regulations are different. They must pay €14.67/metre after 90 days, and must obtain a formal transit log.

There is also a long-standing flat charge of €7.34 when re-launching after being lifted out. Many yards absorb this charge.

NB:The charges introduced by the Greek government in January 2000 for yachts cruising in Greek waters have now been withdrawn for EU registered yachts.

Vessels from other EU countries no longer need a transit log and cannot buy duty free fuel. Transit logs are needed by non-EU vessels and these entitle the holder to purchase duty free fuel.

Navigational aids

Except in major shipping areas, there is little buoyage. Lights are sparse and often low powered. Cruising in this area requires careful perusal of charts and pilots since hazards are not necessarily marked. It should be noted that local datum must be used for GPS or large errors will be encountered. In many cases Greek spelling or Greek script of place names and navigation aids leads to confusion when referring to non-Greek publications.

Inland waterways

There are three waterways in Greece where special rules of navigation are in force:

The Corinth Canal. Designed to reduce the length of the voyage from Italian ports to Piraeus and the Eastern Mediterranean, this ship canal, 4M long and with a depth of 8 metres was opened for traffic in 1893. The canal authority is the state-owned Corinth Canal S.A.

As ships may not pass each other in the canal, permission to proceed must first be obtained by VHF Ch 11 from the canal authority at either end. Canal dues are paid at the eastern end. At all times, comply with the flag and light signals which are clearly displayed at each end of the canal.

Corinth Canal dues are divided into categories depending on the size and purpose of the vessel. Yachts carrying fewer than 25 passengers are in category ST. There is a fixed charge plus a charge related to the yacht's length.

Pilotage is not compulsory for vessels under 800 tons. Normally, all craft in this category proceed under their own power, but tugs are available. In 2005 the charge for an 11m yacht, one way, is €100.

The Evripos Channel. These narrows, which separate the Island of Euboea from the mainland, are crossed at Halkis by a sliding bridge. At times, a current of up to 8 knots flows through the narrows so that the bridge is only opened for shipping when tidal and weather conditions are favourable. This is normally at slack water and the bridge is only opened in the middle of the night to avoid disruption to road traffic. In 2005, the charge for a vessel up to 50 tonnes is €12 plus 25% night supplement and 75% Sunday supplement plus VAT at 18% on total charge.

The Lefkas Canal. A canal separating the Island of Lefkas from the mainland has existed since classical times but the present ship canal and the long, northern breakwater were completed in the last century. Some 3M long and dredged to a minimum of 6 metres this provides a useful shortcut. At the northern end there is an opening bridge, the west end opens every hour on demand for yachts.

Currently north-going traffic goes first. Do not tow in the canal without prior permission. Towing of dinghies is accepted.

ENTRY
EU regulations apply.

Ports of entry
The list of 52 official ports of entry published by the National Tourist Organisation of Greece in *Yachting Greece* include a number which are not thought to have facilities for clearing in foreign yachts. The list which follows is not complete, but is believed to include ports familiar with handling foreign yachts.

West coast

Argostoli (Cephalonia – Ionian)

Katakolon (Peloponnese)

Kerkyra/Corfu (Corfu – Ionian)

Levkas (Ionian)

Patras (Gulf of Patras)

Preveza (Ionian)

Pylos (W Peloponnese)

Vathi (Ithaca – Ionian)

Zakynthos/Zante (Ionian)

Elsewhere

Ayios Nikolaos (Crete)

Alexandroupolis (N Greece)

Chania (Crete)

Corinth (Gulf of Corinth)

Ermoupolis (Syros)

Glifada (Athens)

Iraklion (Crete)

Itea (Gulf of Corinth)

Kalamata (Peloponnese)

Kavala (N Greece)

Khios (Khios)

Kos (Kos)

Lavrion (Saronic Gulf)

Mirina (Limnos)

Mitilini (Lesvos)

Navplion (Argolic Gulf)

Pithagorion (Samos)

Rhodes (Rhodes)

Thessaloniki (N Greece)

Volos (N Greece)

Vougliagmeni Marina (Saronic)

Zea Marina (Saronic)

Entry by road

The normal passport regulations for visitors entering, staying in or leaving Greece also apply to those accompanying a boat and trailer. The width of the boat must not exceed 2.5m otherwise a special police permit may be required; the overall height of the boat on the trailer is restricted to 4m and the maximum combined length of the towing vehicle and the boat on the trailer is 15m. The speed limit on Greek toll roads is 100kph (62mph); 80kph is the rule on other roads, and in towns it is 50kph unless otherwise indicated on road signs. These limits also apply to cars towing a boat on a trailer or with a boat on the roofrack. Commercial vehicles carrying a boat are subject to the speed limits in force for the particular class of vehicle.

Pleasure craft (any small motor, sail or rowing boat) owned by non-EU residents whether on a trailer or roofrack will be permitted to enter Greece duty-free for four months – extendable on application to Customs. The boat will be entered on the owner's passport at the frontier and the owner will not be permitted to leave the country without the boat unless special arrangements are made with Customs.

In June 1996 the following list of crossing points with 24 hour Customs Offices was published by The Automobile and Touring Club of Greece:

Doirani, Euzoni, Niki, Promahonas, Ormenio, Kakavia, Kastanies, Kipi.

Customs

EU regulations apply.

Note that Customs continue to be interested in whether a vessel is carrying drugs, firearms or scuba diving equipment, the latter because diving is forbidden in certain areas.

Documentation

of vessel

Ship's registration papers. The Small Ships Register does not include reference to tonnage nor can it be adapted or modified to do so.

Vessels from other EU countries no longer need a transit log and cannot buy duty free fuel. Transit logs are needed by non-EU vessels and these entitle the holder to purchase duty free fuel.

of crew

Valid passports.

Greek regulations state 'A skipper's licence or other documentation of nautical qualifications and experience are required for pleasure boats under the Greek flag according to the size and type of vessel. For instance a speedboat licence is required for small fast-going vessels and for larger vessels reaching speeds above 25 knots, irrespective of other professional seamanship qualifications. Skippers of yachts under foreign flag should hold equivalent qualifications, issued by their home authorities or nautical clubs'.

International Certificate of Competence (ICC) must be held. It should cover the type of vessel concerned.

Greek insurance regulations

The Greek authorities are now enforcing more stringent third party insurance requirements:

- at least €293,470 liability for death or injury caused by collision, sinking or any other cause, both for those on board and third parties
- at least €146,735 liability for damage
- at least €88,041 liability for sea pollution

A Greek language certificate of third party insurance must be carried on board, showing the amounts in figures, together with the original policy document. Yachtsmen should invite their broker to confirm that they issue such certificates and that the cover includes all stated liabilities.

Dutiable stores

EU regulations apply.

OTHER INFORMATION

The unit of currency is the Euro.

Tel. code from the UK: 00 30

Tel. code to the UK: 00 44

The power supply in Greece is 50Hz 220V.

It is illegal for a non-Greek vessel to tow another vessel within the jurisdiction of a harbour.

Greek authorities have occasionally levied fines for yachts flying torn or worn Greek courtesy flags and for dinghies not carrying safety equipment. This includes lifejackets and flares even in a rubber dinghy setting out on a swimming trip.

Scuba diving is prohibited in most Greek waters, but is allowed in certain areas provided that detector instruments are not used and fishing is not undertaken. Local enquiries should be made.

In order to fish in Greek water you must have an amateur fishing licence.

It is advisable (but not yet compulsory for private yachts) for all yachts to have holding tanks or biological treatment plants. Tanks may not be discharged closer than 6M from the nearest coast. Great care should be exercised when taking diesel on board to avoid spillage. Sea toilets should not be used in harbours. A small spillage of any kind will be very obvious and could result in a substantial and instant fine.

Chartering

Cruising in Greek waters has become so popular in the last 10-15 years that chartering has developed from a small-scale occupation to an industry, which now offers over 2,000 craft to the cruising yachtsman. Many are based in the Athens-Piraeus area, but there are some sailing from Rhodes, Corfu, Thessaloniki and some other islands in the Aegean and Ionian Seas.

It is advisable to cover any informal loan of a boat with a formal written authority from the owner (which should be "notarised" in some way by a solicitor), to avoid the risk of the loan being treated as a formal (and possibly illegal) charter by the Port Authorities. Proof of VAT payment must be carried on board. Company-owned boats must be covered by two formally registered documents, the first permitting use of the boat, the second confirming the authority of the signatory to the first document.

In theory any EU-registered vessel can now legally be chartered in Greece, but the vessel must pass a very stringent, and possibly obstructive, examination by the Greek authorities.

Anyone wishing to do so should apply to the Greek Ministry of Merchant Marine.

Fuel and stores

Following Greece's entry into the EU the availability of spares and materials has greatly improved. The previously endless and expensive process of getting spares through Customs has been normalised, and there are well-stocked chandleries in Corfu, Piraeus and Levkas.

Mechanical and boat-building repairs and licensed liferaft servicing to a high standard are also available in Athens/Piraeus, Levkas, Lavrion, and elsewhere.

Diesel is readily available, as is Camping Gaz. Water is usually available but may be in short supply in the islands, which often have to rely on tanker delivery in the summer.

General provisions including meat, fish, vegetables and fruit are usually available at about the same price as in the UK.

Weather forecasts

There is good Navtex reception from Kevkyra (Corfu K), Heraklion (Crete H) and Limnos (L). Greek TV broadcast a weather chart at 2130. HF/SSB broadcast four times daily.

Publications

British Admiralty charts cover all the coasts and islands.

Greek charts are available from the Hellenic Navy Hydrographic Service.

Mediterranean Pilot Vol III (NP47) Ionian Sea and Gulf of Corinth.

Mediterranean Pilot Vol IV (NP48) Aegean Sea.

Ionian Pilot. Heikell (Imray) 1996.

Greek Waters Pilot. Heikell (Imray) 8th edition 2001

The Blue Guide – Greece (A & C Black).

Greece Yachting - Hellenic Tourism Organisation from the National Tourist Organisation of Greece

Useful addresses

Greek Embassy
1A Holland Park, London W11 3JP
Tel: 020 7221 6467

Maritime Affairs Section - Embassy of Greece Maritime Consular
Tel: 020 7727 0326   Fax: 020 7727 0509

National Tourist Organisation of Greece
7 Conduit Street, London W1R 0DJ
Tel: 020 7734 5997
www.gnto.gr

Automobile and Touring Club of Greece (ELPA)
2/4 Messogion, Athens 115 27
Tel: 748 8800 Fax: 778 6642

British Embassy, Consular Department
Plutarchou Street, Athens 106 75
Tel: Athens 7236 211.

Periandros (This is the Corinth Canal Company)
Kyra Brisi, Korinthians
Tel: 2741030880

British Admiralty Chart Agents
85 Akti Miaouli,185 38, Piraeus
Tel: 4291181

New Company of Corinth Canal
Ithmia
Tel: 0741 37700.

Hellenic Navy Hydrographic Service
Admiralty Building, Klafthmonos Square, 2, Paparigopoulou St, Athens
Tel: 2104183134

Port Police Directorate (for entry by sea)
Maritime and Tourism Section, 150 Gr. Labraki Street, 18518 Piraeus
Tel: 2104191700.

TURKEY

CRUISING

Turkey enjoys a variety of climates from the temperate Black Sea region to the continental climate of the interior and the Mediterranean climate of the Aegean and Mediterranean coastal regions. The coastline of Turkey's four seas is more than 4,000M in length.

Apart from the peak holiday period of July and August, it is not difficult to find quiet and secure anchorages in what is one of the best cruising grounds in the Mediterranean.

The Lycian coast
from Marmaris east to Antalya (about 180 miles).

The Carian coast
from Bodrum south and east to Marmaris, including the Gulf of Gökova and the Datça Peninsula (about 120 miles).

The Ionian coast
from Kusadasi south to Bodrum, including the Gulf of Güllük (about 80 miles).

The Aeolian coast
from Ayvalik south to Kusadasi (about 180 miles).

Istanbul
From Istanbul south to Ayvalik, including the Sea of Marmara and the Dardanelles (about 220 miles).

Harbours and marinas

These are excellent licensed marinas where a yacht may be left unattended, including Atakoy (Istanbul), Kalamis (Fenerbahce), Ayvalik, Golden Dolphin (Cesme), Kusadasi, Bodrum, Marti (Hisaronu), Marmaris, Gocek, Finike, Kemer and Antalya (Setur).

Navigational Aids

Buoyage and lights are rare. Hazards may not be marked, and cruising in these waters requires careful study of charts and pilot.

ENTRY

The Q flag should be hoisted.

Entry by road

There are several places in Italy and Greece from which car ferries run to Turkey. Details are available from the Turkish Tourist Office in London and many travel agents. There is also a land route direct to Turkey but the later stages can be tedious and it may be thought the Balkan area could be hazardous.

Cars, minibuses, caravans and motorcycles can be brought into Turkey for 3 months. These vehicles will be registered in the owner's passport and this registration is cancelled when the owner leaves the country. The period of 3 months can be extended by another 3 months, but 6 months in any one calendar year is the maximum. After that the vehicle should be taken out of the country or left in a Customs bond area (marinas do not usually have vehicle bond areas). Whilst there is a valid permit for the vehicle the owner can leave it in a marina and sail away, but if he wishes to visit another country from Turkey without the vehicle he should take it to the nearest Customs Authority (Gümrük Mudurlugu) so that

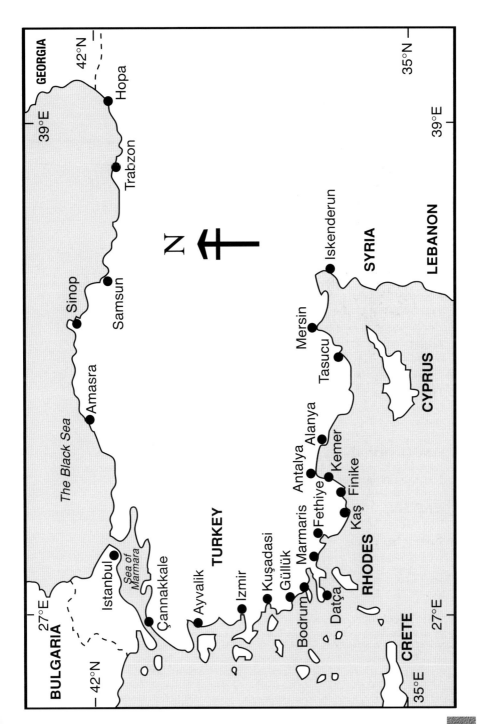

the registration of the vehicle in his passport may be cancelled and the vehicle kept in the customs bond area.

Any towed boats will also be registered in the owner's passport on entry into Turkey. They will be treated as vehicles and subject to the 3/6 months time limits. However if the owner completes a transit log (see below) for them the passport registration will be cancelled and the boat considered as a cruising boat, and, as in the case of yachts, can be kept in Turkey (in a licensed marina) for up to 5 years, provided the boat is used at least once every two years.

There are no limitations on bringing bicycles into Turkey.

Ports of entry

Yachts should enter at a recognised port of entry. Istanbul and Canakkale are the only useful ports of entry for yachts in the Sea of Marmara area (the others are commercial harbours). The ports of entry on the Aegean and Mediterranean coasts south of Canakkale are: Ayvalik, Dikili, Izmir, Cesme, Kusadasi, Güllük, Bodrum, Datça, Marmaris, Fethiye, Kas, Finike, Kemer, Antalya, Alanya, Anamur, Bozyazi, Tasucu (Silifke), Mersin and Iskenderun.

Insurance. A motorist should have either:

a) Green Card international Insurance, endorsed for Turkish territory both in Europe and Asia, or

b) Turkish third party insurance, which can be obtained from any of the insurance agencies at the frontier ports.

In case of an accident, whether or not persons are injured, the police should be notified as a report is essential.

Customs

Anyone planning to take a yacht to Turkey should make careful enquiries about the latest regulations, because these change from time to time.

Visiting yachts require a Transit Log, valid for 365 days and renewable thereafter. A Transit Log form must be purchased (often from a marina office) for the equivalent of US$30. and then stamped by the Health Authority, Passport Police, Customs Patrol and Harbourmaster in that order.

When the yacht leaves Turkish waters the Transit Log must be surrendered on departure and a new one obtained on re-entry. The log must be kept on board when the yacht is left in a marina for laying up if the captain / skipper leaves Turkey for another country. The Transit Log remains valid until the original 365-day period expires or until the yacht leaves Turkish waters.

The Transit Log will include your declaration of equipment on board, which will include a dinghy and outboard, and electronics. In theory the boat can be checked on departure to ensure that the gear is still there, and has not been illegally sold. In practice this is seldom if ever enforced, but there has been the occasional problem when an item has been stolen, since technically duty then becomes payable.

More serious questions will be asked about firearms and about diving equipment, the latter because diving is forbidden in a number of areas to protect archaeological treasures: the export of these is strictly forbidden. The yacht is liable to be impounded if this law is contravened.

Documentation

of vessel

- Ship's registration papers, Certificate of Insurance, Ship's Radio Licence.

of crew

- UK citizens require visas, obtainable on entry for £36 or from the Turkish consulate in London at a cost of £10. An appointment with the consulate can be made online at www.turkishconsulate.org.uk. They are valid for multiple entry for 90 days and can be renewed on expiry. Liveaboards and their crew can apply for residence permits for the term of their berthing contract in a licensed marina. The possible taxation implications should be investigated
- International Certificates of Competence are required for skippers.
- The Transit Log includes a crew list. No other document is needed. In principle, crew changes should be reported and the Transit Log amended.

OTHER INFORMATION

Tel. code from the UK: 00 90

Tel. code to the UK: 00 44

Banking hours are 0830 -1200 and 1300 -1700 (not Sat or Sun).

The unit of currency is the Turkish lira which has recently been reformed, so that one New Lira replaces an old lira unit with a face value of 1 million. Old currency will be legal tender until the end of 2005.

The Turkish courtesy flag should be flown at all times, and it should be in good condition.

The coast is under surveillance and visitors should refrain from removing any antiquities from the coast or coastal waters, as the penalty is the confiscation of the yacht.

Although holding tanks are not yet compulsory for private yachts they are virtually a necessity, as any discharge of any kind may be considered illegal. One yacht was fined £1,000 recently for discharging in harbour. You are in tideless waters and often anchored in places where you want to swim. Although the rules may seem to be harshly applied they are sensible. Harbours where one needs to be especially careful are Bodrum, Bozburun, Gocek (Town Quay), Kalkan and Kas. Caution should also be exercised with Bilge water.

There are facilities in the marinas to have holding tanks pumped out from the shore. Alternatively you can pump out at sea but you should be at least three miles offshore.

Chartering

Crewed yachts based on traditional local design (gülets) are available at a number of ports for charter. With modest sail area and powerful diesel, they are very suitable for local conditions. Bareboat and skippered yachts are also widely available for charter. There are also numerous UK based charterers who advertise in yachting magazines.

Fuel and stores

Spares are not difficult to obtain in the marinas, but if not available there or in a local town chandlery they may be delivered, mostly within a day, from the main distributor in (usually) Istanbul. If parts have to be imported there can be considerable delays (Customs procedures can be elaborate). Antifoulings and general chandlery are available at most marinas. Engine repairs and most general repairs can be carried out at the major marinas all of which have travel-lifts. Diesel and water are readily available at most harbours. Camping Gaz is very difficult to find, but Turkish gas has identical fittings and is obtainable everywhere. General provisions, fruit and vegetables are in good supply, as is fresh meat and fish. Also many different frozen foods.

Weather forecasts

There is good reception of Navtex forecasts from Iraklion, Limnos and Cyprus. There are also Navtex stations at Istanbul and Izmir. Some coast radio stations (eg Antalya) carry weather bulletins in Turkish and English.

Publications

BA charts for the coast are suitable, but have not been surveyed recently; Turkish charts are also available.

Admiralty Publications

Black Sea Pilot

Mediterranean Pilot Vol IV

Mediterranean Pilot Vol V

Turkish Waters Pilot. Heikell (Imray).

Turkey's Turquoise Coast. Heikell (NET)

Turkey - A Travel Survival Kit. Brosnahan (Lonely Planet)

Useful Addresses

Turkish Embassy
43 Belgrave Square, London SW1
Tel: 020 7393 0202

Turkish Tourist Office
170/173 Piccadilly, London W1V 9DD
Tel: 020 7629 7771 Fax: 020 7491 0773
www.tourismturkey.org

Turkish Maritime Lines
Alternative Travel, 146 Kingsland High Street, London E8 2NS
Tel: 020 7923 3230

Turkish Consulate
Rutland Lodge, Rutland Gardens, Knightsbridge, London SW7 1BW
Tel: 020 7591 6900 Fax: 020 7591 6911
turkishconsulate@btconnect.com
www.turkishconsulate.org.uk

THE REPUBLIC OF CYPRUS
(Member of the European Union)

CRUISING

Cyprus is the third largest island in the Mediterranean and enjoys a mild climate with an average 340 days of bright sunshine each year. Summer winds are steady and, in winter, it is unusual for the sea and air temperatures to drop below 16°C and 9°C respectively.

Medical services and supplies are excellent.

Since July 1974 Cyprus has been divided by the Green Line patrolled by the UN. The northern sector is controlled by Turkey and is known as the Turkish Federated State of Northern Cyprus. It is not formally recognised by any country except Turkey. The southern sector, which is Greek speaking, is known as the Republic of Cyprus and is universally recognised. The Republic of Cyprus will not allow yachts which have called anywhere in Turkish held territory to enter any Republic harbour. They hold a blacklist of yachts.

Yachts may, however, proceed directly to and from the Republic of Cyprus and mainland Turkey.

Northern Cyprus

Northern Cyprus is not a member state of the European Union and has fewer tourist facilities and is relatively unspoilt compared with the Republic of Cyprus.

The Greek language names which appear on charts and maps have been changed to Turkish names. Thus, for example, Nicosia is now Lefkosa, Famagusta is Gazi Magusa and Kyrenia is Girne.

Gazi Magusa is the main commercial port of the north, but mooring facilities for yachts are poor; there are slipways but little else.

The small town of Girne on the north coast is 15M from Nicosia and only 45M from Turkey. It is a holiday resort with a small picturesque harbour. There is also a small commercial harbour with simple marina facilities, including hard standing. Entry fees are very reasonable but there is limited room for visiting yachts. There are no repair facilities and no chandlery. Diesel can be delivered to the quayside from a filling station about 200m from the harbour.

Yachts entering Northern Cyprus are required to fly the special Northern Cyprus courtesy ensign.

There are a number of attractive anchorages on each side of Gime, but many are restricted by the military, and yachts may be asked to move.

Republic of Cyprus

The notes in the following sections refer only to the Republic of Cyprus.

Harbours and marinas

Larnaca marina has full facilities. Situated in the centre of the town, it is very crowded, reservations 9-12 months ahead are needed for long stays.

In Limassol there is very little room for yachts in the old commercial harbour which has become almost entirely a fishing harbour. St Raphael's marina has full facilities, and is 20 minutes bus ride out of Limassol.

Paphos harbour, on the west coast of the island, is picturesque and has had some development. There is little room for yachts, but it is possible to anchor or moor with a long line ashore.

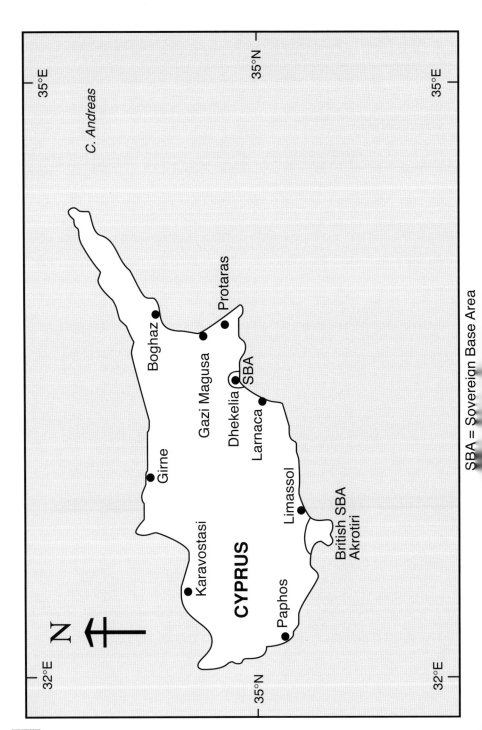

N

C. Andreas

Boghaz

Protaras

Gazi Magusa

Girne

Dhekelia
SBA

Larnaca

Limassol

Karavostasi

CYPRUS

British SBA
Akrotiri

Paphos

SBA = Sovereign Base Area

32°E

35°E

35°N

ENTRY

Ports of entry

Larnaca, Paphos, St. Raphael Marina, Limassol.

Entry by sea

No yacht may enter the Republic of Cyprus through Northern Cyprus ports or touch at any point on the area controlled by Turkey. According to the Laws of the Republic of Cyprus, entry into the Turkish controlled areas of the island is illegal. Vessels entering those ports are liable to be arrested when within the waters of ports under the control of the Cyprus Government. Entries are closely monitored and a fine of up to 10,000 Cyprus pounds and/or up to six months imprisonment is imposed on any transgressor. All yachts must clear in and out of each port. Landing cards are issued together with form C104 (temporary importation). This form is issued for six months and entitles the holder to import duty free equipment for the yacht. A total of one year temporary importation is allowed before duty must be paid on the yacht.

When entering Cypriot waters a yacht should fly the Cyprus flag.

Cyprus Radio maintains continuous listening watch on VHF Ch 16. In an emergency, you would be transferred to Cyprus Marine Police on Ch 16.

NB The Cyprus Marine Police may approach your yacht when you are sailing and ask for details of your passage and number of persons on board.

It is advised that, unless approaching a port of entry, vessels should maintain a distance of 500m offshore by day and 1,000m by night.

Customs

Remain on board until clearance has been given by the Marina Attendant, Marine Police, Customs Officer, Immigration Officer and Health Inspector. Passports will be retained by Immigration. A Form C104, valid for six months, is issued by Customs.

Documentation

of vessel

- Ship's registration papers, which should be presented to the port authorities at the port of entry. Evidence of insurance may be requested.
- VAT certificate. An official document is essential - you could face heavy fines without it.

of crew

- Valid passports. Crew lists (five copies) should be made available at the port of entry. Two passport-size photographs are required for gate passes.

Dutiable stores

Consumable stores are available 24 hours prior to departure, spirits being limited to one case per person.

Duty free tobacco and liquor on board should be declared on entry and may be removed and retained by the Customs until departure when it will be returned. Duty free tobacco and liquor may be obtained in all ports, where there are bonded stores.

OTHER INFORMATION

Tel. code from the UK: 00 357

Tel. code to the UK: 00 44

The unit of currency is the Cyprus pound (CYP) divided into 100 cents. Cyprus money is readily accepted in the Turkish area but the Republic of Cyprus will not accept Turkish lira.

During the summer all shops close from 1300 to 1600 and all government offices close for the day at 1330. Bank opening hours are 0830-1200 Monday to Saturday.

Weather forecasts

Only from coastal radio stations or Greek National broadcasts (see Greek section). BFBS radio gives forecasts on the hour for coastal waters. FM 95.5m or 98.9m. RAF Akrotiri gives 24hr weather Tel: 00 357 2596 6577

Good Navtex forecasts can be received from Limnos, Heraklion and Cyprus.

Fuel and stores

Good facilities and diesel are available at Limassol and Larnaca (which has a travel-lift).

Chartering

Contact one of the marinas or JMP Luxury Yacht Cruises, PO Box 4875, Nicosia, Cyprus.

Publications

BA charts -2074 Cyprus -775 Paphos -776 Kyrenia -796 NE Coast -850 Limassol 851 Larnaca-Famagusta.

Admiralty Sailing Directions, Mediterranean Pilot Vol V.

The Eastern Mediterranean. Denham.

Turkish Waters Pilot & Cyprus. Heikell (Imray).

Useful Addresses

High Commission of the Republic of Cyprus
93 Park Street, London W1K 7ET
Tel: 020 7499 8272

Cyprus Government Tourist Office
17 Hanover Street, London W15 1YP
Tel: 020 7569 8800

Thesea Savva (Admiralty Chart Agents)
118 Franklin Roosevelt Avenue, Limassol, Larnaca Marina
Tel: 00 357 4653 110 / 653 113   Fax: 00 357 4624 110

Larnaca Marine
Tel: 00 357 2465 3110/653 113
Fax: 00 357 2462 4110

St Raphael Marina Limassol
Tel: 00 357 2563 5800
www.visitcyprus.org.cy

Cyprus Tourist Office
Nicosia: Tel: 00 357 2233 7715

SLOVENIA - CROATIA - MONTENEGRO
(Member of the European Union)

CRUISING

This eastern Adriatic area boasts one of Europe's most indented and beautiful coastlines. There are over 700 islands and almost everywhere the mountains drop steeply to the sea, the scenery is magnificent and the water generally very clear. There is good cruising in the small section of the Slovene coast but it is Croatia that provides the largest cruising area. The whole coastline and all the islands of the three countries are now completely open and welcoming to visiting yachts. Formalities are simple and speedily dealt with at all ports of entry.

The major cruising areas are:

Slovenian coast, Istria, The Kornati National Park, Islands South of Split to Dubrovnik and Gulf of Kotor (Montenegro)

SLOVENIA

Harbours and marinas

There are three marinas along the 32km coast: Portoroz, Izola and Koper all with full facilities and well protected. The harbour of Piran is also suitable for short/medium length stays but gets crowded in mid-summer.

Note: Anchoring is prohibited in three Protected Areas and two Fishing Reserves.

Information is available locally.

ENTRY

Ports of entry

Ports of entry: Koper and Piran - year round 24hrs, Izola May - Oct 0800 - 2000.

Report arrival to customs/police usually in the same administrative building. An annual 'use of aids to safe navigation' fee may be charged - dependent on vessel length.

Prior to departure one is obliged to inform the customs/police; ensure all marina fees are paid before reporting departure - these documents may be asked for.

Slovenia joined the EU in 2004.

Entry by road

Contact your own insurance company regarding cover as each one treats the area differently, some issue green cards, some don't. Third party insurance is probably available locally. A valid driving licence and the vehicle's original registration papers should also be carried.

Documentation

of vessel

* Original documents for the vessel (Part 1 Registration or SSR).
* Proof of ownership or authorisation for its use.
* A crew list.

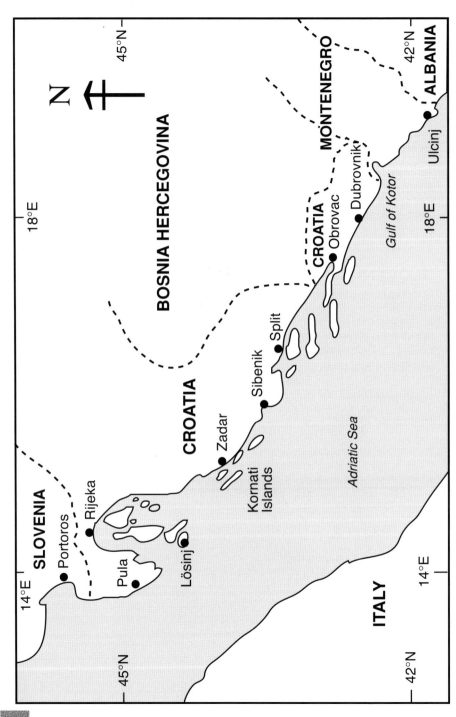

of crew
- Passports.
- Captain's Certificate of Competence (eg ICC).
- VHF radio licence.
- Visas are not required.

Equipment
There is a required minimum equipment regulation: a foreign vessel must have at least:
- an anchor of suitable weight with at least 30m of rope or chain
  a mooring rope at least 10m long - two auxiliary paddles - regulation lights
- auxiliary bilge pump - first aid kit - 6 hand flares - mirror (for water skiing)

OTHER INFORMATION
Telephone code from UK 00 386

Important phone numbers: Police 113   Ambulance 640-0980

The national currency is Slovene Tolar (SIT) with approx. 350 to £1 (in Spring 2005)

Banks open: 08.30-12.30/14.00-16.30 Mon-Fri: 08.30-12.00 Saturday.

Post Offices open 08.00-18.00

Cash points can be found and credit cards are frequently accepted in larger shops and restaurants.

Voltage: 220   Water: Drinkable

Health centres offer medical and dental services in all three municipal centres (Koper, Izola and Piran).

Chartering
Chartering may only be conducted with a Slovene registered company. It is a criminal offence to rent vessels from an unregistered company.

Fuel and stores
Fuel is available in the marinas and Piran. A good selection of chandlery is also available.

Weather forecast
Rijeka   VHF 24   0535, 1435, 1935 UT Croat/English

Trieste VHF 25   0135, 0735, 1335, 1935 UT Italian

VHF 68 Continuous Italian/English

Satellite maps and synopses posted on marina notice boards.

CROATIA
Harbours and marinas
Marinas - Adriatic Croatia International Club (ACI) operate 22 marinas and there are at least 20 more privately run, all with full facilities.

Harbours - Many harbours have pull-off lines to their ground tackle, at others moor bow or stern-to own anchor. Water and electricity often available.

Anchorages - Countless quiet unspoilt bays. Ensure you are well dug in and a clear exit is available, sudden strong winds (Bora) can occasionally occur.

Cost - Marina prices are quite expensive but they depend on length of stay and time of year. Discounts are occasionally available - ask. Harbours charge a nominal fee dependent on facilities and popularity of the area. Charges for anchoring are levied in the National Parks and if you pick up a buoy, these are laid in only a few places.

NB check ground tackle is suitable for your boat size.

A daily tourist tax is also due when paying for these facilities.

July/August are the most crowded months with many Austrian, German and British charterers and Italian visitors.

ENTRY

Ports of entry

Arrival must be at a port of entry which is listed in various almanacs and pilot books. Customs and police are often housed in the same building or the harbour master will phone them to visit your vessel.

Authorities are courteous and helpful and are usually only interested in firearms or drugs.

An annual cruising permit (vinjeta) must be purchased, issued by the harbour master and valid for 12 months from date of issue. The cost is approx. £135 and this allows one to sail in and out of the country at any time. Report departure to police/customs and the back of the permit will be completed. Keep the permit in a safe place if a return within 12 months is contemplated.

The number of persons shown on the cruising permit list of persons may not exceed double the number of persons the craft is allowed to carry + 30%. The full text of the regulation can be found at www.mmtpr.hr (select English, then Sea, then Nautics).

Entry by road

Contact your own insurance company regarding cover as each one treats the area differently, some issue green cards, some don't. Third party insurance is probably available locally. A valid driving licence and the vehicle's original registration papers should also be carried.

Documentation

of vessel

- Ship's registration papers.
- Cruising permit with crew list attached (updated at any crew change).
- Crew list.
- Certificate of Insurance.

of crew

- Passports.
- Captain's Certificate of Competence (eg ICC).
- Visas are not required.

OTHER INFORMATION

Telephone code from UK 00 385

Important phone numbers: Police 92   Fire Brigade 93 Ambulance 94

National currency is the Kuna (100 lipa) approx. 10 to £1 (Spring 2005). Banks and Post Offices are generally open 07.00-19.00 Mon - Fri and 08.00-13.00 on Sat. Many POs keep longer hours during the summer. All major credit cards are accepted in larger shops and most restaurants and larger towns have cash points.

Medical care is available in hospitals providing a 24hr emergency service.

Voltage: 220   Water: Drinkable

Weather forecast

Riyeka VHF 24   0535, 1435, 1935 UT. Split VHF Ch 07, 21, 28, 0545, 1245, 1945 UT.
Dubrovnik VHF Ch 07, 04, 0625, 1320, 2120 UT. All Croatian/English.

Internet site: http://meteo.hr/index_en.html

Forecast in Croatian, English, Italian and German: http://prognoza.hr/prognoze_en.html

Satellite maps posted at marinas

Chartering

There are at least 11 charter companies operating flotilla and bare-boat holidays based in various marinas.

Fuel and stores

Diesel and petrol are freely available. Few chandlers but marina and charter fleet workshops can be helpful. Sailmakers are few and far between.

MONTENEGRO
ENTRY

Ports of entry

Arrival must be at a port of entry. Melijine (in north) or Bar (in south). Customs, police and harbour master either come on board or must be visited; the crew must stay on board until signed in.

Entry by road

Contact your own insurance company regarding cover as each one treats the area differently, some issue green cards, some don't. Third party insurance is probably available locally. A valid driving licence and the vehicle's original registration papers should also be carried.

Documentation

of vessel
• Ship's registration papers, Insurance and crew list.
• An annual cruising permit has to be purchased, the cost approx. $US65.

of crew
• Passports, Certificate of Competence (captain).
• Visa not required.

OTHER INFORMATION

Euro widely accepted: credit cards rarely accepted.

Publications

Admiralty charts available for the whole area at various ratios.

The Croatian Hydrographic Office produce charts (1:100,000) of the whole coast.

Admiralty Sailing Directions - Mediterranean Pilot Vol. 3

Adriatic Pilot. T&D Thompson (Imray)

Navigational Guide to Adriatic - Croatian Coast (English) Lexicographical Institute, Zagreb

Mediterranean Cruising Handbook. Rod Heikell (Imray) 2005-2006 edition

Mediterranean Almanac

Useful Addresses

Croatian National Tourist Board
2 Lanchesters
162-164 Fulham Palace Road
London W6 9ER
Tel: 020 8563 7979 Fax: 020 8563 2616
E-mail: info@cnto.freeserve.co.uk
Web site: www.croatia.hr (Very full information pack on request)

Embassy of the Republic of Croatia
18-21, Jermyn Street
London SW1Y 6HP
Tel: 020 7434 2946   Fax: 020 7434 2953

Slovenian Tourist Board
The Barns, Woodlands End
Mells, Frome, Somerset BA11 3QD
Tel: 0137 3814233 Fax: 0137 3813444

Embassy of Slovenia
10 Little College St
London SW1P 3ST
Tel: 020 7222 5400 Fax: 020 7222 5277

Cyprus High Commission Yugoslav Interests Section
5, Lexham Gardens
London W8 5JJ
Tel: 020 7370 6105   Fax: 020 7370 3838

National Tourist Organisation of Montenegro
Stanka Dragojerica 26
81000 Podgorica,
Montenegro
Tel: 00 381 81 41591/45959

UK Embassy Croatia
Vlaska ulica 121
HR-10000 Zagreb
Croatia
Tel :+385 1455 5310 Fax: +385 1455 1685

MALTA
(Member of the European Union)

CRUISING

The Republic of Malta comprises the islands of Malta, Gozo and Comino. These low, arid, densely-populated islands situated midway between Europe and Africa are still of great strategic importance, as they have been over the centuries, and their history is both colourful and fascinating.

Malta is a convenient staging point for yachtsmen on passage in the central Mediterranean and a popular destination for those wishing to over-winter afloat or lay-up their yacht ashore. It has extensive facilities for yachts, easy communications and is an interesting, though small, cruising ground in its own right with picturesque harbours and attractive anchorages. There is a good live-aboard community around Marsamxett Harbour with regular quizzes, book-swaps and other social events. English is one of two official languages and is widely spoken.

Harbours and marinas

The principal yachting port is Marsamxett Harbour on the north side of Valletta. The harbour is divided into three main creeks; Sliema, Lazaretto and Msida. There are yacht berths in Msida Marina and on both the north and south sides of Lazaretto Creek. The outer entrance to the harbour is open to the north-east and strong winds from this direction, known locally as a gregale, send a swell rolling in. The berths in Msida Marina are reasonably well protected but those in Lazaretto Creek can be badly affected and a yacht moored there should not be left unattended while a gregale is blowing. There are no berths for yachts in Sliema Creek which can be dangerous in a gregale.

The berths in Msida Marina and on Ta'Xbiex Quay on the south-west side of Lazaretto Creek are administered by the 'Malta Maritime Authority'. Their offices, known as the 'Yachting Centre', are situated on Msida Point at the entrance to Msida Marina. Berths are allocated as they become available on a 'first come, first served' basis. They cannot be booked in advance either personally or through an agent. The greatest pressure is during September and October when visitors start to arrive for the winter whilst the permanent berth-holders still have their boats in the water. During these months berths for visitors may be unavailable or restricted to a few days but when the permanent berth-holders start to lift out in November, space becomes available and there is usually plenty of room for those who wish to over-winter afloat.

Malta Maritime Authority does not provide pick-up lines on Ta'Xbiex Quay though some berths do have lines left behind by previous occupants. If staying for a few weeks or longer many yachtsmen employ a diver to attach a line to the heavy ground-chain that runs parallel with the shore. Those not doing so lie to their own anchor.

The facilities on the Manoel Island shore of Lazaretto Creek have recently been taken over by a new company known as 'Manoel Island Marina'. They have already built two pontoons running out from the shore and three more are planned for the near future. The company intends to build a breakwater to shelter their berths from the gregale but no time-scale has been stated.

There is a small marina at Mgarr on the island of Gozo and an interesting harbour at Marsaxlokk in the south of Malta. A new marina known as 'PortiMaso' with approximately 100 berths has been built in St Julian's Bay as part of the expansion of the Hilton Hotel.

Extensive facilities for laying-up ashore are available on Manoel Island. The principal facility, 'Manoel Island Yacht Yard', is very popular and advance booking is recommended. It has

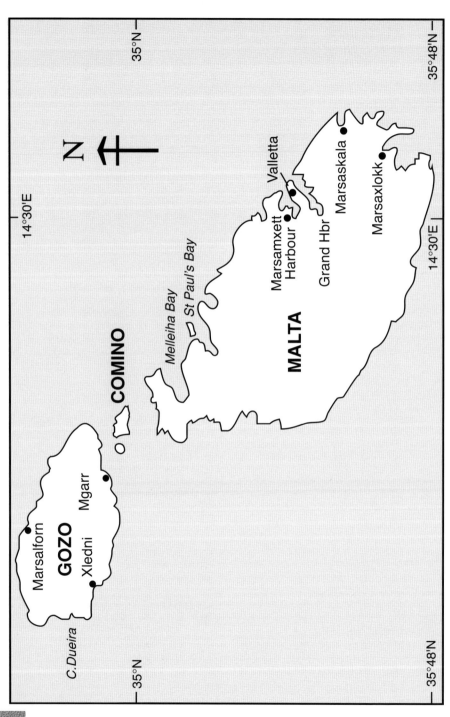

two travel hoists, a crane and seven slipways for vessels up to 500 tons. Security in the yard is good. 'Manoel Island Marina' has its own lay-up facilities. It currently lifts boats with a mobile crane but a travel hoist is planned.

There have been plans for some time to build a 'Super-Yacht' Marina in Grand Harbour but work has not yet been started.

ENTRY

Ports of entry

The principal port of entry for yachts is Marsamxett Harbour but, between 16th June and 30th September, clearance in and out can also be made at Mgarr on Gozo.

Customs

Yachts arriving from abroad should contact Valletta Port Control on VHF Channel 12 when within range for entry instructions. Yachts arriving during office hours [0800 to 1200 and 1300 to 1700 (1900 during the summer)] are usually directed to the Customs office at the Yachting Centre at the entrance to Msida Marina. A short section of the quay behind the marina wall is reserved for yachts seeking clearance. The formalities are simple and usually take no more than 10 minutes.

Yachts arriving outside office hours are directed to clear inwards in Grand Harbour. This is a commercial harbour with no provision for yachts and mooring near the Customs office can be difficult. Yachtsmen are strongly advised to time their arrival to enable them to clear inwards at the Yachting Centre.

Yachts and pleasure craft may be kept in Malta without liability for tax if their registered owners are non-resident foreigners, if the boats are exclusively intended for use by the owners or their authorised representatives (who must also be non-resident foreigners) and provided that the boats are not chartered out. Tax-free yachts and pleasure craft are entitled to tax-free spares.

Documentation

The Department of Customs requires only a Certificate of Boat Registry for the vessel and valid Passports for every member of the crew. A number of forms have to be completed when clearing in but these are simple and normally present no problems. UK citizens do not need Entry or Transit Visas. There are no restrictions on crew changes. The master of a departing vessel must present a receipt from the Malta Maritime Authority showing that all dues have been paid.

Before departure from Malta, whether by sea or by air, crew members must present themselves to the Customs and Immigration officials at the Yachting Centre where their passports will be stamped. It is particularly important to remember to do this before going to the airport. If and when the crew fly back to Malta, their passports will be 'date-stamped' at the airport. This procedure grants entry for three months, after which time they have to go to the Port Police in Floriana to have their passports re-stamped. This does not apply to crew who remain on the island having entered by yacht since their passports will not have been 'date-stamped' on entry.

Quarantine regulations

Yachts with cats or dogs on board that have Certificates and Ear-Chips are allowed to berth alongside after the animals have been inspected by the Health Department Vet. However, yachts with uncertificated animals on board may not berth alongside at any time. Further information can be obtained from the Port Health Department. Telephone: +356 2122 4810.

Dutiable stores

Duty-free stores and fuel can be obtained by making arrangements with one of several agencies for completion of the necessary forms. 24 hours notice is required for fuel and up to 48 hours should be allowed for stores, which will be delivered under Customs supervision. Customs require yachts to leave within 24 hours of embarking duty-free stores, which may not be consumed within territorial waters.

OTHER INFORMATION

Maltese telephone numbers now have 8 digits. Add 21 in front of old six-figure numbers.

Telephone code from the UK: 00 356 (no area code is required within Malta).

Telephone code to the UK: 00 44   Overseas Operator: 194

Police: 191   Ambulance: 196   Fire Brigade: 199

The unit of currency is the Maltese lira (Lm) which is divided into 100 cents. Cash Machines are widely available. There is no limit to the amount of foreign currency visitors may bring into Malta, providing it is declared upon arrival. However, the maximum amount of Maltese currency that may be brought into Malta is Lm 50. Visitors may not take out of Malta more than Lm 25 in Maltese currency.

Electricity is 240V single phase, 50Hz. Sockets are the same as in the UK.

Vehicles drive on the left-hand side of the road. There is a speed limit of 64 kph (40mph) on highways and 40kph (23mph) in urban areas. Public transport is cheap and efficient.

A reciprocal health agreement gives UK citizens free medical and hospital care for visitors staying less than one month. Yachtsmen staying for a longer period have to pay some of the costs of treatment so may wish to take out suitable insurance.

Malta keeps Central European Time (GMT +1). Daylight Saving Time (GMT + 2) is kept from the last Sunday in March until the last Sunday in October.

Chartering

Details can be obtained from the Valletta Yacht Club. Telephone: +356 2133 1131.

Weather forecasts

Malta Radio transmits daily weather forecasts in English at 0803, 1203, 1803 and 2303 local time on 2625kHz and VHF 04 after preliminary calls on VHF 12. A Navtex transmitter gives forecasts for Malta and the surrounding waters within a 50 mile radius.

Fuel and stores

Fuel is available from an anchored barge near the entrance to Msida Marina and a small road tanker tours the berths in Msida Marina and Lazaretto Creek. Camping Gaz and Calor Gas bottles can be re-filled at one of the chandlers.

There are many small shops and two large supermarkets within walking distance of Lazaretto Creek. The supermarkets stock many imported goods from the UK that are not normally obtainable in the Mediterranean and they deliver to the quayside free of charge. There are numerous chandlers and spares of all types are readily obtainable. There are several internet cafes and a launderette along the seafront between Manoel Island Bridge and Sliema. Vans selling vegetables and/or fish can be found parked in strategic points around the towns on Malta. A few such vans visit the quays each day.

Drinking water is produced on Malta by de-salination. Though it is said to be of good quality when it leaves the plant, it is often contaminated at the point of delivery as it passes through old rusty iron pipes. Water and electricity at the yacht berths on Ta'Xbiex Quay are metered and charged for and new connections cannot be made there either during the evenings or weekends. However, water and electricity in Msida Marina are included in the price for berths, and can be used at any time.

There are many services available for yachts in Malta that can be difficult to obtain elsewhere in the Mediterranean with the added advantage of communication in English. Manoel Island Yacht Yard has extensive workshops for engineering and repairs of all kinds.

Agents

There are many Yacht Agents operating in Malta, one of the largest being S & D Yachts Ltd. For a fee they will act on your behalf in locating goods and services but use of them is not compulsory.

Publications

BA Chart 194 covers Malta and there are also harbour charts.

Admiralty Sailing Directions

Mediterranean Pilot Vol 1

Ports and Anchorages Handbook (Royal Malta YC)

Italian Waters Pilot. Heikell (Imray)

Mediterranean Almanac. Heikell (Imray)

North African Pilot. RCC (Imray)

Useful Addresses

Malta High Commission
Malta House, 36-38 Piccadilly, London W1J 0LE.
Tel: 020 7292 4800   Fax: 020 7734 1831

Malta Tourist Office
Unit C, Park House, 14 Northfields, London SW18 1DD.
Tel: 020 8877 6990   Fax: 020 8874 9416
Website: www.visitmalta.com   E-mail: info@visitmalta.com or office.uk@visitmalta.com

Malta Maritime Authority
Yachting Centre, Msida Marina, Ta' Xbiex, MSD 011.
Tel: +356 2133 2800   Fax: +356 2133 2141
E-mail: charlesaxiaq@mma.gov.mt or chris.schembri@mma.gov.mt

Customs Office
Yachting Centre, Msida Marina, Ta' Xbiex, MSD 011.
Tel: +356 2133 5691   Fax: +356 2133 9187

Manoel Island Marina
Manoel Island, Gzira, GZR 06.
Tel: +356 2133 8589   Fax: +356 2134 1714
Website: www.manoelislandmarina.com   E-mail: info@manoelislandmarina.com

Manoel Island Yacht Yard
Manoel Island
Tel: +356 2133 4453/4454   Fax: +356 2134 3900
E-mail: info@yachtyard-malta.com or miyy@global.net.mt

State Hospitals
Malta: +356 2124 1251   Gozo: +356 2156 1600

S & D Yachts Ltd
57 Gzira Road, Gzira, Malta.
Tel: +356 2133 9908   Fax +356 2133 2259
The address for mail for yachts berthed in Marsamxett Harbour should take the form:
Yacht-Name, Msida Marina (or Ta' Xbiex Quay), The Yachting Centre, Ta' Xbiex Seafront, MSD 11, Malta.

ALBANIA

CRUISING

It is advisable to check with the Foreign and Commonwealth Office for the latest advice before arrival as detailed regulations are difficult to obtain.

No visas are necessary for EU passport holders, but a US$10 entry tax and a US$10 exit tax must be paid.

ENTRY

Ports of entry

Durres and Saranda. Entry tax of approx. $US57 is levied.

Visiting yachts are dealt with as commercial ships and the tax and any harbour dues are paid via a shipping agent who also adds his fee making the whole deal expensive. Clear in and out of each port.

$US and Euro are widely accepted: credit cards and travellers cheques are not.

Advice is to drink bottled water and use UHT milk.

Publications

Admiralty Sailing Directions - Mediterranean Pilot Vol.3

Adriatic Pilot. T&D Thompson (Imray) New Edition 2000

Mediterranean Cruising Handbook.

Rod Heikell (Imray) 2005/2006

Mediterranean Almanac 2001/02

Useful Addresses

British Embassy
Rruga Skenderberg 12, Tirana, Albania
Tel: 00 355 423 4973/4/5   Fax: 00 355 424 7697

Saranda Travel Agent:
Spiros Angjeli
Tel: 00 355 732 4398 Fax: 00 355 732 3380

THE BLACK SEA

CRUISING

The Black Sea is a viable cruising area, but weather patterns are more demanding than the Mediterranean, with occasional storms, long fetches and heavy seas. Distances between ports of call are in many cases significant: from the Bosphorus northwards to Odessa is approximately 315 nm and from Constanta eastwards to Batumi is some 570 nm.

In 1997, a Black Sea yacht rally was sponsored by Ataköy Marina, and in 1999 it was extended to all six coastal countries and has done much to ease the way for visiting yachtsmen.

With the Danube open to maritime traffic it is again possible to reach the Black Sea via the inland waterways of Europe. Access is also possible from the Russian inland waterways, which are now open to pleasure craft. However, the majority of yachtsmen will sail from the Aegean to Istanbul and then northwards against the current up the busy Bosphorus - a rewarding passage easily completed in one day; there is a good overnight anchorage at Poyraz on the east bank at the northern end.

Navigational aids

GPS is the only electronic aid available. The Bosphorus is well-lit and buoyed, as are major harbours around the coast.

Navtex

Mariupol B

Odessa C

Istanbul D

Varna J

TURKEY

(See page 49 for visa and transit log requirements)

Plentiful spares should be bought in Istanbul before setting out.

Yachts should clear out at Karaköy in Istanbul, and at the same time buy a Transit Log for re-entry, since Ports of Entry on the Northern Turkish coast do not hold stocks of this document. When northbound, Igneada, to the W of the Bosphorus, is not a Port of Entry, being only a small fishing port, but yachts may moor there providing they have previously bought a Transit Log. Southbound it is technically possible to clear in at Hopa, Trabzon, Giresun, Samsun, and Sinop, but in practice a yacht may be sent on from harbour to harbour until it reaches Istanbul.

There are many safe harbours along the coast, where visiting yachts are a rarity, and likely to be welcomed with typical Turkish hospitality. The unspoiled nature of the area means that facilities are limited and a smattering of the Turkish language is desirable. At Trabzon a yacht may moor alongside by the Coastguard building in the commercial port or in the unfinished marina; Samsun has a sailing club within the large commercial harbour; Sinop has space for yachts within the fishing port on the S side of the peninsula; at Amasra a yacht may anchor in the inner harbour. Most other harbours are fishing harbours, but there is always space for a yacht to moor up stern- or bow-to, with the help of friendly fishermen.

Water and fuel are usually obtainable in jerrycans, but a minitanker for fuel can be arranged in some ports.

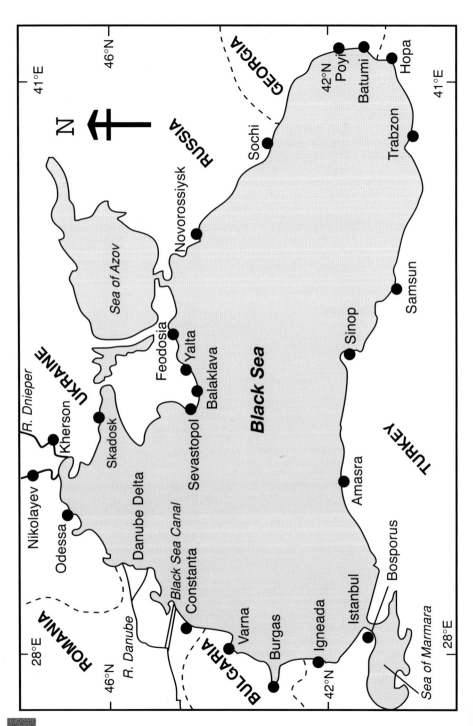

BULGARIA

Visiting yachtsmen do not need visas, but passports are stamped in and out at each Port of Entry. Sailing Permission is issued by the harbourmaster to sail to the next Port of Entry, and when leaving Bulgaria a Certificate of Clearance is issued for presentation in the next country. Usual ship's papers are required, and Certificates of Competence have been demanded. Located on the western Black Sea coast, bounded by Turkey in the South and Romania in the North. There are several developed summer tourist resorts with fine sandy beaches, but boating is not developed. The population is about 8 million and the capital is Sofia. The cruising area is from the Turkish border to Kavarna with no suitable harbours north of here. Some new marinas are under construction.

ENTRY

Ports of entry

There are three Ports of Entry: Balchik, Varna and Bourgas.

At Bourgas Customs/Border Police will visit the yacht on arrival. No-one should go ashore until formalities have been completed. Bourgas is recommended; since it will issue a Temporary Navigation Certificate (in exchange for Ship's Papers and a fee of US$30) permitting free passage along the attractive coast from Nesebar to Aktopol on condition that each night is spent in one of six designated harbours. The yacht must return to Bourgas to obtain a Certificate of Clearance and the Ship's Papers.

At Varna, where there is a yacht club within the commercial harbour, Customs/Border Police will visit the yacht on arrival. No-one should go ashore until formalities have been completed. On departure the harbourmaster will issue Sailing Permission after payment of fees, a prerequisite for stamping out by Passport Control.

At Balchik a yacht must clear in with Customs/Border Police (which do not operate at weekends) and harbourmaster.

At Nesebar, a secure and picturesque harbour, there is a small yacht club where yachts are very welcome.

Documentation

of vessel

- Ship's registration papers
- Certificate of insurance
- Ship's stamp (very useful but not essential)

of crew

- Passport. The passport must be valid for at least three months after the end of the intended stay. A visa is not required for passport holders from the following countries and permission to stay will be given for 30 - 90 days depending on the country:

    All European – 30 or 90 days or no visa required

    Australia, Canada, Israel, Japan, New Zealand, United Kingdom, USA – 30 days

    Chile – 90 days

    Korea and Tunisia – no visa required

    For all other countries a visa is required

- International Certificate of Competence (or similar national qualification)
- Crew list (varies from 1 to 7 copies)
- Declaration that no firearms, narcotics or other dangerous substances and no stowaways are on board
- Declaration of all provisions, spirits and cigarettes on board

OTHER INFORMATION

Telephone code from the UK : 00 359
Telephone code to the UK : 00 44
Ambulance: 150 Fire and emergency safety services: 160 Police: 166
On the coast there is almost total coverage for mobile phones.
The unit of currency is the leva.

Fuel and stores

All fuel has to be obtained from garages and transported in containers.
Adequate shops, bars and restaurants in most towns. Ship chandlers in Varna and Bourgas

Navigation Hazards

Inshore many fixed fishing nets and mussel farms, mostly only marked by small plastic
bottles. Lights sparse and sometimes non-operational.

ROMANIA

Visiting yachtsmen with EU passports do not need visas, but passports are stamped in and
out at each Port of Entry by Frontier Police. A Clearance Permit is issued by the
harbourmaster covering the voyage to the next port or country.

Customs/Immigration and harbourmaster will visit the yacht, and the usual ship's papers are
required. On departure, clear out with the same officials.

Romania has only a short coastline S of the Danube Delta, with limited possibilities for
cruising, but the Sulina arm of the Danube is the main navigation route and an international
waterway. To cruise in the Delta a permit is required which is issued in Tulcea.

The principal port is Constanta, where a yacht should clear in. Here there is a major area of
commercial docks which should not be entered by a visiting yacht, but there is a separate
yacht harbour at Port Tomis below the old town where a yacht may lie alongside. It is
possible to leave a yacht unattended and visit Bucharest by train, as it is at Mangalia, where
there is also a yacht harbour. At Sulina, at the entrance to the Danube canal, it is possible to
moor alongside, respecting the 4 kt seaward current. Yachts en route to or from the Ukraine
via the Danube Canal should clear in/out at Tulcea, which is a Port of Entry.

Harbours and marinas

Mangalia, Port Tomis (north of Constantia) and Sulina.

Documentation

• Usual ship's papers

• Passports with at least six months validity. Romania is visa free for 90 days for passport
  holders from (amongst others) the EU, USA, Canada, Norway and Switzerland. It is visa
  free for 30 days for passport holders from most East European countries in the former
  Soviet Bloc.

Customs

Passports are stamped in and out at each port by Frontier Police who will visit the yacht as
well as the other authorities (Customs/Immigration and harbourmaster). A Clearance Permit
is issued by the harbourmaster covering the voyage to the next port or country. On
departure, clear out with the same officials.

OTHER INFORMATION

Telephone code from UK: 00 40
Telephone code to UK: 00 44
Ambulance: 961 Emergency hospital: 962 Police: 955 Fire: 981 International emergency calls: 971

On the coast there is almost total coverage for mobile phones.

The unit of currency is the lei. Currency may only be changed at an official change bureau or bank. Before leaving the country change lei back into dollars.

Fuel and stores

Fuel has to be obtained from garages and transported in containers, except in the Danube delta where there are fuel barges and in Port Tomis where a tanker lorry can visit the boat.

Navigation Hazards

The river Danube brings down vast amounts of silt, and depth near the mouths constantly changes and can be totally different from those shown on the charts.

There are many fixed nets marked by small plastic bottles.

UKRAINE

With a coastline of 900M, from Mariupol to the Danube delta, Ukraine offers good cruising with shelter to be found each night in commercial harbours or isolated anchorages without the need for night passages.

Harbours and marinas

Within the commercial harbour at Odessa there is a full-blown marina with pontoons and satisfactory facilities, including a fuel jetty. There are good moorings in the Dnieper delta and there is good shelter at Skadosk commercial harbour. Sevastopol is a naval port, but there are several mooring possibilities on the south side of the harbour, including the Yacht Club Yug, the Russian Navy Yacht Club, the Yacht Club Sevastopol, and Ushakova Balka. There is a new yacht marina with some facilities at Balaclava, and at Yalta (Massandra) there is also a small yacht harbour with some facilities inside the commercial harbour. Otherwise there are a number of anchorages along the coast.

Ports of entry

Feodosia, Yalta, Sevastopol, Yevpatoria, Skadosk, Ocakov, Odessa and Izmail.

When 12 miles off call LEBED (coastguard) on Ch 16, and give yacht name, flag and numbers on board with their nationalities. LEBED will ask:

Do you speak Russian?

Your position

What do you want?

Why do you wish to enter the country?

Switch to working channel.

On arrival at the first Port of Entry a yacht should request a Customs document that covers all the ports to be visited. This may take some time. A Decree was passed in September 2002 stating that foreign yachts may clear in on arrival in Ukraine and clear out only when leaving the country: it will no longer be necessary for the yacht to clear in and out at every port.

Visas must be registered within three days of arrival.

Documentation

Visitors must obtain a visa in advance from the Ukrainian Consulate in London or with the assistance of Ataköy Marina in Istanbul. In Istanbul a visa normally takes four days to issue, or two days express. Cost varies with length of validity: in 2000 an express visa for two months cost US$100. Since May 2000 visa applications no longer need to be supported by an invitation from Ukraine. Passports must be valid for six months after the expiry date of the visa. State health insurance must also be purchased (in 2000 two months cost US$56). Although UK citizens are technically exempt, this is not recognised at Embassies. Private health insurance is not adequate.

The usual ship's papers are required. A ship's stamp is a necessity for use on all official papers, showing boat name, register number, port of registry and name of owner.

A General Declaration for Customs should be prepared before arrival, as well as a good number of crew lists.

Coastguard tracking

LEBED tracks yachts by radar along the coast and requests contact every time the yacht moves, normally on Ch 16. Information will be given about bombing practice and closed areas.

OTHER INFORMATION

US dollars are the most useful currency to bring with you, but local currency – the grivna – is obtainable from ATMs with Visa or Mastercard, which are also accepted by shops in the larger towns.

Fuel and stores

Fuel (and water) will need to be carried in jerrycans except in Odessa. It is advisable to carry a number of fuel filter elements, and there are very few chandlers for other spares. Food shopping is excellent and cheap, with a market in every town or village, and provision shops replacing the old-style Soviet supermarkets.

RUSSIAN FEDERATION

A visa is required, to be obtained in advance. An application for a visa must be accompanied by an invitation to visit the country. Each port is treated as a new country so a multiple entry visa is necessary if intending to visit more than one harbour. Some difficulties with officials have been reported, since they are not familiar with the concept of privately-owned cruising yachts wishing to cruise their coastline.

At Novorossiysk, there is a yacht marina with pontoons and some facilities, including an engineering and repair shop. At Sochi, there is a yacht club with all facilities, but entry can be refused. It may be found useful to employ an agent.

The unit of currency is the rouble.

GEORGIA

A visa is required, to be obtained in advance in the country of residence. However, "urgent entry" visas can be obtained at very high cost in Poti, or more reasonably from the Georgian Consulate in Trabzon (Turkey). Normal ship's papers are required.

Poti is the only Port of Entry. Customs, immigration and harbourmaster will visit the yacht on arrival. There is a Yacht Club at Poti, but no special facilities for yachts at Batumi.

The unit of currency is the lari.

Publications

Cruise the Black Sea - Doreen and Archie Annan - Ataköy Marina 2001

Admiralty Sailing Directions – Black Sea

Turkish Waters Pilot – Rod Heikell – Imray

Black Sea Cruising Guide – Rick and Sheila Nelson – Imray

BA Charts for the area are suitable and Turkish charts provide reasonable cover.

Useful Addresses

Bulgarian Embassy
186 Queen's Gate, London SW7
Visa information 0900 117 1208 (premium rate)   020 7584 9400

Romanian Embassy
4 Palace Green, London W8 4QD
Visa information 0900 188 0828 (premium rate)   Consular Section 020 7937 9667

Ukraine Consulate
78 Kensington Park Road, London W11 2PL
Visa information (premium rate) 0900 188 7749   020 7243 8923

Romanian National Tourist Office
83a Marylebone High Street, London W1
0900 555 8860 (premium rate) 020 7224 3692
www.romaniatourism.com

Russian Embassy
5 Kensington Palace Gardens, London W1
Visa information 0900 117 1271 (premium rate)   020 7229 8027

Russian National Tourist Office
167 Kensington High Street, London W8 6SH   020 7937 7207

Georgian Embassy
3 Hornton Place, London W8 4LZ
Visa information 0900 160 0558 (premium rate)   020 7937 8233

Ataköy Marina
Istanbul Fax: 00 90 212 560 72 70   E-mail: marina@atakoymarina.com.tr

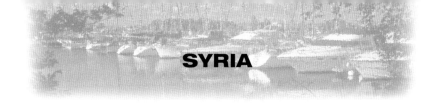

SYRIA

CRUISING

Although the short 175 km coastline has many beaches under forested mountains, there are no natural harbours and only four artificial harbours – at Lattakia, Baniyas, Tartous and Ruad. In 2000, a new marina at Lattakia was opened, the Syrian Yacht Club, with modern facilities for 25-39 boats up to 40m LOA. It is 15 km from the airport. Otherwise the purely commercial ports are without facilities for yachts and there is no scale of fees for berthing, port services, etc. As a result, a yacht visiting those ports is likely to be charged several hundred dollars for a stay of a few days, without water, electricity or any other facility.

The language is Arabic but French and to some extent English is widely understood.

The unit of currency is the Syrian pound (S£) divided into 100 piastres.

US$ are commonly used and are extremely useful.

Tel: code from the UK: 00 963   Tel: code to the UK: 00 44

ENTRY

Ports of entry

Yachts may not visit Syria if Israeli stamps are on crew passports.

Arrival should be made preferably at Lattakia, in daylight and at 90° to the coast. ETA must be reported when 12 miles west of the port. Visiting yachts are not permitted to cruise along the coast and navigation at night is not recommended in view of the risk of being taken for a hostile vessel.

Formalities have been reported as complicated. Yachts planning to visit Syria are recommended to try and arrange for the services of a local agent beforehand.

Documentation

of crew

- Valid passports and visas.

- Visas can be obtained in London or on arrival in which case extra passport photographs will be required. Passports should be carried at all times when ashore since security checks are frequent.

- An international driving licence is required if driving in Syria.

Publications

BA charts numbers 2532 and 2633 cover the Syrian coast: 1036 and 2796 give harbour plans.

Admiralty Sailing Directions

Mediterranean Pilot Vol V

Useful Addresses

The Syrian Embassy
8 Belgrave Square, London SW1X 8PH   Tel: 020 7245 9012
There is no Syrian Tourist Office in London, but the Syrian Interest Section at the above address may help.

Syrian Yacht Club
P.O.Box 2503 Lattakia - Syria
Tel: 00963 041 474146   Fax: 00963 041 222379   E-mail: syrychtclb@mail.sy   VHF 9, 16

LEBANON

CRUISING

Although there is still tension in the border area between Lebanon and Israel, Lebanon is essentially a peaceful country with good facilities for visiting yachtsmen, at least at Jounieh, a relatively affluent suburb of Beirut.

Jounieh Marina is modern, well equipped and hospitable. The nearby town has good shopping and banking facilities, and the interior of the country has great scenic variety and historic interest.

ENTRY

Ports of entry

Sailing in territorial waters is permitted 24/24 hrs. Beirut and Tripoli are official ports of entry for commercial vessels only. It is advisable and less expensive for yachts to head first for Jounieh, where foreign yachtsmen are welcomed and where neither formalities nor security present a problem. The procedure for entry is to contact Jounieh Yacht Harbour on VHF Ch 16 or11 when 20nm offshore on a bearing of 270° from Jounieh. The marina manager will inform the authorities of your arrival and your ETA. Yachts arriving from Israel will be denied entry. An Israeli stamp on a crew passport will preclude entry.

On arrival at Jounieh Yacht Harbour berth temporarily at the fuel station just inside the marina for formalities to be completed. There is a fee of US$58 for harbourmaster and customs clearance and of US$50 for immigration clearance, but there are no mooring fees for the first three days.

There is a new exit tax for each person leaving Lebanon by air or yacht. It is US$24 per person if going to Cyprus and US$40 per person for every other destination.

Documentation

of vessel

• Ship's registration papers.

• Letter of authority if the owner is not on board.

• Clearance from last port showing reasonable date of departure for Jounieh.

of crew

• Valid passports, and visas which can be obtained on arrival. However, for visits of only one week, shore passes will be given on arrival to holders of passports issued in the US, the EU and in other European countries (except for citizens of Turkey and of countries formerly in the Soviet Bloc who should obtain visas in their own countries before entering Lebanon).

• Crew list.

OTHER INFORMATION

Tel. code from the UK: 00 961

Tel. code to the UK: 00 44

Telephone calls to the UK can be made through the operator from the PTT in the town.

French and (to a lesser extent) English are widely spoken.

The unit of currency is the Lebanese pound.

US$ notes are acceptable in most shops and restaurants. Other currency is freely exchanged at banks and change shops. Travellers cheques are grudgingly accepted at some change shops but not at banks.

Fuel and stores

Diesel and petrol are available without formality at the fuelling berth just inside the marina entrance.

There is a yacht chandler near the marina gate and several good supermarkets in the town. Cash can be obtained with the more common credit cards through a variety of banks.

Weather forecasts

Weather forecasts can be obtained daily from the marina office.

Publications

British Admiralty Charts and Sailing Directions are adequate.

Useful Addresses

Lebanese Embassy, Consular Section
21 Kensington Palace Gardens, London W8 4RA
Tel: 020 7229 7265

Automobile & Touring Club du Liban
PO Box 115 - Jounieh - Lebanon
Tel: 00 961 9 932 020 or 640 220 Fax: 00 961 9 932 468 E-mail: atclmarine@terra.net.lb

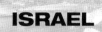

ISRAEL

CRUISING

Israel's coastal waters have little to offer cruising yachts, but many of those who find themselves at this end of the Mediterranean may want to visit the tourist sites. English is widely understood and spoken.

Harbours & marinas

Tel Aviv Marina has excellent security and modern facilities but is somewhat expensive and usually crowded. It also has a very difficult entrance from the sea, and entry should not be attempted with onshore waves. The marina will provide a pilot free of charge if requested by VHF.

The marina in Haifa harbour is run by a club, but visitors are welcome. Shelter is excellent, and the pontoons can be reached in all weathers. The road entrance is far from the town centre.

There are marinas at Herzlia, Ashdod and Ashkelon. Both Herzlia and Ashkelon are substantial marinas equipped with travel hoists. Herzlia is emerging as the major yachting centre of Israel.

The harbours of Acre and Jaffa accommodate yachts, but not visitors.

Navigational Aids

Haifa and Tel Aviv are well lit but the navigational lights merge with the city lights and can be difficult to recognise.

ENTRY

Ports of entry

Haifa, Herzlia, Tel Aviv and Ashkelon.

The Q flag should be flown on approaching Israeli waters, and listen on VHF Channel 16 from a distance of 50 miles or less. At not less than 25 miles from shore, report particulars to Haifa Radio 4XO. They will ask a list of obvious questions, including position, course, speed, ETA and passport details of crew.

Interception by a Navy vessel should be expected. At night a searchlight will illuminate the yacht (with a loaded machine gun pointing at it!). It is recommended to switch off the autopilot while in the close vicinity of the Navy vessel, since the Naval electronics have been known to interfere with the autopilot function. The same list of questions will again be asked, and instructions might be given.

It is obligatory to continue listening on Channel 16 unless requested by Haifa or the Israeli Navy to change to a working channel. When within 12 miles of shore, the yacht's speed should not exceed 15 knots.

Customs

Haifa provides 24hr service, and the officials will come to the boat. Follow the Police patrol boat guiding you to a mooring.

Herzlia and Tel Aviv officials usually work marina office hours which are from 08:00 till 17:00hrs. Check this with the marina before arrival. Yachts arriving outside these times might be requested to stand off the marina. If in doubt, ask the intercepting Navy boat for advice.

Arrival at the Ashkelon Marina must be coordinated by the marina management to ensure that officials are available on arrival.

Clearance is free of charge. The crew may not leave the yacht until clearance is completed.

Documentation

of vessel

- Ships registration papers
- Third party risk insurance (for the marinas)
- Crew list

of crew

- Valid passports. Visas are not required by British passport holders. Passports are normally stamped on entry, but on request the police will stamp a separate sheet of paper to prevent difficulties when visiting other countries.

Departure

for Israeli destination

Check out at marina office and ask for details of any active firing practice areas or closed security areas on proposed route. Once out at sea, radio the Israeli Navy to tell them of proposed route.

for foreign destinations

Give 12 hours notice of departure. Check out at marina office and get a marina exit permit (and get details of any closed security areas or active firing practice areas on proposed route). The police then stamp and return the crew passports at the marina and the yacht may leave. Out at sea radio the Israeli Navy to tell them of proposed route.

OTHER INFORMATION

Tel. code from the UK: 00 972

Tel. code to the UK: 00 44

The unit of currency is the Shekel

Banking Hours are 08:30 – 13:00 daily except Saturdays, and 16:30 – 18:30 Sunday to Thursday.

Fuel and stores

The range of goods available in the shops is similar to that found in most western countries, although prices tend to be slightly higher. Most towns have supermarkets, but fresh produce will be cheaper in the markets.

Fuel berths for yachts exist in Herzlia, Tel Aviv and Ashkelon. Fuelling without a car is a problem in Haifa. Chandlery shops are located in or near Herzlia and Tel Aviv marinas, and also in Haifa city and Ashdod town.

Publications

BA chart number 2634 covers the coast and 1585 and 1591 give harbour plans.

Admiralty Sailing Directions, Mediterranean Pilot Vol. V.

Useful Addresses

Israeli Embassy
2 Palace Green, London W8 4QB
Tel: 020 7957 9500

Israeli Government Tourist Office
180 Oxford Street, London W1
Tel: 020 72991111
"Sailing News" web site gives detailed information ranging from shipping forecast to chandlery addresses. A visit to this site is a must for anyone heading to Israel.
www.sailing-news.co.il

Ashdod Marina
PO Box 14282, Ashdod
Tel: 088557246 Fax: 088556810

Ashkelon Marina
PO Box 5335, Ashkelon
Tel: 086733780 Fax: 086733823 www.ashkelon.co.il

Herzlia Marina
PO Box 5881, Herzlia
Tel: 099565591 Fax: 099565593 www.herzliya.co.il

Jaffa Marina
PO Box 49, Old Jaffa Port
Tel: 036832255 Fax: 036830377

Tel Aviv Marina
PO Box 16285, Tel Aviv
Tel: 035272596 Fax: 035272466 www.telaviv-marina.co.il

Haifa Marina
PO Box 33539, Haifa
Tel: 048422106

Acre Marina
PO Box 1086, Acre
Tel: 049919287 Fax: 048258382

EGYPT

CRUISING

The Mediterranean coastline consists of a long stretch of sandy beaches. There is very little shelter and the coast is mostly exposed to breakers and northerly winds.

Harbours and marinas

Alexandria has a western and an eastern harbour, each protected by a breakwater. The eastern harbour is recommended for visiting yachts; it has a designated anchorage area for yachts and small craft, with fairly good holding.

Port Said lies at the northern end of the Suez Canal, and a berth may be found at the Port Fouad Yacht Club or the anchorage nearby. There is very heavy commercial traffic at Port Said.

Inland waterways

Suez Canal

The procedure for transiting the Suez Canal is quite complex and very time-consuming unless an agent is employed. The Felix Maritime Agency (Nagib Latif) specialises in assisting foreign yachts to pass through the Canal and operates in accordance with a published price list.

Use of an agent is strongly recommended and this could avoid unpleasant difficulties. Requests for gifts should not necessarily be refused.

River Nile

A yacht should only attempt navigation of the Nile subject to the following requirements:

– a strong hull to withstand stone banks and passing barges

– a powerful engine to overcome strong currents

– removable masts

– maximum draft of 1.75m

– reliable echo sounder

ENTRY

Ports of entry

Alexandria and Port Said, or Safaya, Hazghada and Suez if arriving via the Red Sea.

Customs

If an agent is employed, he will normally handle all dealings with the Customs and Immigration authorities. Otherwise, the yacht will be visited by Coastguards and Customs Officials.

Special Customs measures are taken for yachts intending to enter the Nile or the Suez Canal.

Documentation

of vessel

- Ship's registration papers
- Ship's Radio Licence.
- The following documents should be obtained at the port of entry:
  1. Currency transfer receipt
  2. Health Certificate
  3. Security permit (for the River Nile)
  4. Customs list showing the yacht's equipment.
  5. Insurance Policy (for the Suez Canal)
- Any or all of these documents should be shown as demanded by the local authorities, when applying for visa renewal or a departure permit.
- Six copies of the crew list showing surname, forenames, passport number, status aboard (i.e. crew member) and date of birth.

of crew

- Valid passport.
- Entry into Egypt is open to yachts and yachtsmen of all nationalities. Israelis are permitted provided they carry an entry visa previously obtained from the Egyptian Embassy or Consulate in Israel.
- All crew members will require an entry visa, obtainable from Egyptian Embassies and Consulates abroad, or from local authorities on arrival at any port of entry.
- Usually visas are valid for thirty days from the date of issue, an additional fifteen days is permissible provided there are good reasons for the long stay. On expiry, a new visa should be applied for, in which case you may be required to transfer the sum of US$180 per person, or the equivalent, into Egyptian currency. Children under the age of twelve are exempted from the requirements to transfer currency.
- Your entry visa must be registered at the main office of Immigration, Passports and Nationality Administration at the port of entry, within seven days of acquisition. Failure to do so will result in a fine.
- No restrictions are placed on the amount in cash or travellers' cheques carried or transferred, provided it is declared. The transfer or exchange of currency should be made through banks or their branches in certain first class hotels. You are warned not to deal with the black market, however profitable it may appear.

DEPARTURE

Yachts departing from Egypt should do so from a port of entry. A departure permit should be applied for from the Coast Guard Authorities. All permits, documents and currency transfer receipts previously obtained on arrival or transfer should be submitted, together with passports and the crew list, to the Authorities. Any changes in the crew members must be entered on the crew list. Yachts should depart as soon as the departure permit is obtained. However, in case of difficulty such as engine trouble, serious damage, foul weather or absence of favourable winds, departure can be postponed for 24 hours. If the departure is delayed for longer than 24 hours then you will have to apply for a fresh departure permit.

OTHER INFORMATION

Tel. code from the UK: 00 20

Tel. code to the UK: 00 44

The unit of currency is the Egyptian pound divided into 100 piastres.

English and French are widely spoken.

Publications

BA charts numbers 3356, 2574 and 2573 cover the coast.

Numbers 3325, 3326, 3119, 243, 2681 and 2578 provide harbour approaches and plans; 234 and 233 are required for the Suez Canal and approach.

Admiralty Sailing Directions:

Mediterranean Pilot Vol V

Red Sea and Indian Ocean Cruising Guide. Lucas (Imray)

Egypt for Yachtsmen from the Egyptian Tourist Information Office.

Useful Addresses

Embassy of the Arab Republic of Egypt (Consular Affairs)
2 Lowndes Street, London SW1X 9ET
Tel: 020 7235 9777

Egypt Tourist Information Office
170 Piccadilly, London W1
Tel: 020 7493 5283

Egyptair
29 Piccadilly, London W1
Tel: 020 7437 6309

Centralex Marine Horizon
10 Mohamed Ahmed El Afify Street
San Stefano, Alexandria, Egypt
Tel: 03 586 4939

Felix Maritime Agency
PO Box 618, Port Said, Egypt
Tel: 00 20 66 3333132   Fax: 00 20 66 3333510   www.felix-eg.com

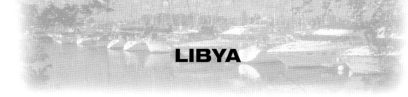

LIBYA

UN Security Council sanctions were lifted in April 1999 and the Foreign & Commonwealth Office advise that safety and security are generally good.

There are strict laws concerning the possession or consumption of alcohol and for public criticism of the country, its leadership or religion. Visitors should on no account attempt to bring alcohol into the country. It is necessary to exercise great sensitivity for local standards and codes of behaviour. Dress should be modest. There should be no public display of affection between individuals. Photography in the vicinity of ports, stations and other public utility installations should be avoided.

British nationals should obtain a visa before travelling to Libya. For information on entry requirements, check with the Libyan People's Bureau, 61/62 Ennismore Gardens, London SW7 1NH Tel: 020 7589 6109. It is unclear, however, whether as in many countries with similar rules, it may be possible for the crews of vessels arriving by sea to be issued with temporary shore passes at the time of arrival.

All vessels navigating in Libyan waters should have serviceable VHF radio equipment and should keep a listening watch on Channel 16 at all times. Port authorities should be contacted on Channel 11, 12 or 16 before arrival, permission is required to move from one Libyan port to another. Movement in Libyan waters is permitted only by day. Refuse and waste water may not be discharged; holding tanks are essential.

Insurance companies may be reluctant to offer cover in this area.

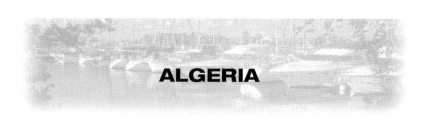

ALGERIA

Although the 750M rugged coastline of Algeria has a number of possible ports and fishing harbours, including a marina at Sidi Fredj, near Algiers, the Foreign and Commonwealth Office strongly advises against visiting the country because the political situation is unstable. There have been numerous murders and armed attacks on foreigners in recent times and yachtsmen are advised to avoid calling at Algerian ports or approaching the coast.

TUNISIA

CRUISING

Tunisia has some 820M of coastline – 650 of them sandy beaches. As a rule a safe berth can be found after a coastal passage of no more than 40 miles. The official language is Arabic, but most Tunisians also speak French.

Tunisia is hotter than countries in the north of the Mediterranean and is at its best in the autumn or spring. Winds are reasonably consistent in direction and strength, but in the spring they often blow from the south, carrying sand which will deposit itself all over the decks.

It is reported that care is required with laid moorings in Monastir Marina due to very strong NW winds which are common in winter.

Anchoring along the coast, especially at night, is forbidden without prior authorisation, however short daylight stops appear to be tolerated. Checks are made by patrol craft.

Tunisians are not allowed to board foreign yachts.

Harbours & marinas

There are six major marinas:-

Tabarka is a fishing harbour with an area of the port dedicated to visiting yachts.

Bizerta, a large commercial harbour near the end of a canal, has a small marina in the outer harbour with guest pontoon.

Sidi Bou Said marina has a travel-lift and limited chandlery.

Tunis, another large commercial port up a canal, has a marina near the entrance at La Goulette; it tends to be full most of the time.

El Kantaoui marina has a travel-lift and visitors berths. It is some distance from shopping facilities although there is a small local supermarket.

Monastir is a large marina with water and electricity, also a supermarket, laundry and many restaurants on site. A separate management runs the travel-hoist. Chandlery suitable for fishing boats is available from hardware shops in the town. The marina is near the town centre and convenient for the airport.

Hammamet - Yasmine Hammamet Marina was inaugurated in 2003 with 740 berths surrounded by apartments, villas, shops and leisure areas. There is a yard with a travel hoist of up to 150 tons. A marina is under construction at Hammamet South.

In addition there are major harbours, including Kelibia, Sousse, Mahdia and Sfax.

Care is needed in many harbours due to silting and the absence of channel markers.

Navigational aids:

There is good buoyage around major ports. For RDF stations see Mediterranean Almanac (Imray).

ENTRY

Ports of entry

Tabarka, Bizerta, Sidi Bou Said, La Goulette, Kelibia, El Kantaoui, Sousse, Monastir, Mahdia, Gabes, Houmt-Souk and Zarzis.

Yachts must report at an official port of entry to Port Police, Harbour Officers, Customs and Frontier Police who will all study yacht and personal documents and stamp them. All personnel must remain on board until formalities have been completed. Passports will be stamped with a three month entry permit which may be renewed for a further three months. Customs will issue a manifeste and the Frontier Police a Déclaration d'Entrée, granting permission to cruise in Tunisian waters for three months. Crew lists may be required both at the initial entry and at subsequent ports of call.

Customs

Customs will require a list of all valuable equipment carried on the yacht. The export of dinars is strictly forbidden, and exchange receipts should be retained in order to facilitate the sale of surplus dinars on departure. Antiques may only be exported by permission of the Ministry of Cultural Affairs.

Documentation

of vessel

- Ship's registration papers. Evidence of ownership of the vessel may be required. In this connection it is important to note that the SSR document on its own does not satisfy this requirement. A bill of sale should also be carried (or a charter party agreement if the yacht is not owned by the persons on board). An insurance certificate, a list of objects of value, and a list of firearms should be carried.
- A crew list may be required at each port of call.

of crew

- Valid passports.
- An International Certificate of Competence is advisable. There are no restrictions on crew changes provided these are notified.
- Visa needed after three month stay.
- Non-EU Citizens may require a visa and they should enquire at the Tunisian Embassy in London beforehand.

Temporary importation

The Tunisian authorities encourage yacht owners to keep their yachts permanently in the country, and the facilities reflect this. Owners leaving their boats in Tunisia to return home by air can obtain a document from Customs which enables them to bring back yacht equipment duty free.

Yachts may be 'immobilised' for the winter by Customs and this period will not count against the six months total navigation period. It is reported that to be granted this concession the owner must first have a contract with the relevant marina. Whilst 'immobilised' the yacht may not be moved without the permission of the Harbour Police.

DEPARTURE

On departure, it is necessary to report to Customs and Frontier Police. If there is no local office, time must be allowed for officials to arrive from the nearest town or airport. The entry documents must be surrendered and passports stamped.

OTHER INFORMATION

Tel. code from the UK: 00 216

Tel. code to the UK: 00 44

The unit of currency is the Tunisian dinar (TND), divided into 1,000 millimes. Dinars may not be imported into Tunisia. Rate of exchange is set by the government. Banking hours are Monday to Friday 0800-1100 in the summer and an additional two hours in the afternoon during the winter.

The crime rate in Tunisia is low. The cost of living is relatively low, half that of London.

Fuel and stores

Fuel is cheaper than in many Mediterranean countries and there are fuel berths at all the main marinas. Water is usually available, and it is possible to have Camping Gaz bottles refilled at Sidi Bou Said, El Kantaoui and Monastir. It is also possible to use Tunisian gas bottles with a Camping Gaz installation. General stores are available in markets and supermarkets. Wine and beer can be obtained, spirits are expensive.

Weather forecasts

Weather forecasts may be obtained from the Harbour Master or by contacting the marine weather centre at the coastal ports of La Goulette, Sfax, Mahdia or Bizerta.

A shipping forecast (in French) is broadcast by Tunis Radio on 1768.4kHz. Forecasts can also be received from Lampedusa (in English and Italian) on 1876kHz and from Malta (in English) on 2624.8kHz.

Chartering

The Tunisian National Tourist Office can supply details of chartering facilities. Cruising yachts and catamarans can be chartered from Tunisia Yachting Loisirs at Monastir. Le Club Nautique de Sidi Bou Said (Tel: 270 689) will advise on local sailing and water skiing.

Publications

BA charts are adequate for cruising in Tunisia. French charts are more detailed and more up to date.

Admiralty Sailing Directions: Mediterranean Pilot Vol 1

Guide to Tunisia. Maurice (McMillan Graham)

North Africa RCC. von Rijn & Hutt (Imray)

Rough Guide to Tunisia (Penguin)

Useful Addresses

Tunisian Embassy
29 Prince's Gate, London SW7 1QG
Tel: 020 7584 8117

Tunisian National Tourist Office
77a Wigmore Street, London W1U 1QF
Tel: 020 7224 5561 Fax: 020 7224 4053
Email: tntolondon@aol.com   Web site: www.tourismtunisia.co.uk

Tunisian National Tourist Office
1 Av. Mohamed V, Tunis
Tel: 341 077

MOROCCO

CRUISING

From the Algerian frontier to the Straits of Gibraltar the sandy coast extends for some 250M with rocky promontories of which Cabo Tres Forcas is the most notable. The vast range of the Rif Mountains rise above the frequent low-lying mists which can develop rapidly into dense fogs.

Harbours and marinas

There are large harbours at Tangier, Al Hoceima and the Spanish enclaves of Ceuta and Melilla and smaller ones at El Jebha, Ras el Ma and M'Diq (which may not be open for yachts). There are marinas at Restinga Smir and Kabila.

ENTRY

Ports of entry

There are no defined ports of entry but yachts are required to report to both Customs and Immigration authorities on arrival and prior to departure. Entry and clearance formalities are in fact required at all ports visited. Customs offices exist everywhere except in the smallest harbours and Port Police will be found throughout.

The Q flag should be hoisted when entering Moroccan waters.

Documentation

of vessel

• Ship's registration papers.

of crew

• Valid passports, but no visas. Crew changes are not restricted. There are reports of entry being refused if Israeli stamps are on crew passports.

Temporary importation

An initial period of three months is permitted.

OTHER INFORMATION

Tel. code from the UK: 00 212

Tel. code to the UK: 00 44

The unit of currency is the dirham (Dh), divided into 100 centimes. Dirhams may not be exported.

Ferries ply from Algeciras to Ceuta and Tangier.

Fuel and stores

There are no facilities for embarking duty-free stores. Fuel and water are usually available. Camping Gaz can be obtained in Ceuta and Melilla.

Drugs

It should be noted that the Moroccan authorities are waging a major campaign against drug smuggling. Yachts are automatically suspect and may be searched at any time. It is best to avoid anchoring or night passages along the coast.

Anchoring is not normally allowed near harbours.

Publications

BA charts Numbers 773 and 2437 cover the coast, and 580 gives harbour plans.

Admiralty Sailing Directions:

Mediterranean Pilot Vol I

North African Pilot. von Rijn (RCC/Imray)

Useful addresses

Moroccan Embassy
Tel: 49 Queens Gate Gardens, London SW7 5NE

Moroccan National Tourist Office
205 Regent Street, London W1R 7DE
Tel: 020 7437 0073

USEFUL CONTACTS

RYA
www.rya.org.uk
0845 345 0400

RYA Cruising
cruising@rya.org.uk
0845 345 0370

RYA Legal
legal@rya.org.uk
0845 345 0373

RYA Training
training@rya.org.uk
0845 345 0384

RYA Technical
technical@rya.org.uk
0845 345 0383

RYA Despatch (book orders)
orders@rya.org.uk
0845 345 0372

Cruising Association
CA House, 1 Northey Street,
Limehouse Basin, London E14 8BT
Email: office@cruising.org.uk
www.cruising.org.uk
www.cruising-association.com
020 7537 2828 (T)
020 7537 2266 (F)

Maritime & Coastguard Agency (MCA)
www.mcga.gov.uk
023 8032 9100
Email: infoline@mcga.gov.uk

**Marine Accident
Investigation Branch (MAIB)**
www.maib.dft.gov.uk
023 8023 2527 (24 hours)

HMSO
www.hmso.gov.uk
0870 600 5522

HM Revenue & Customs
www.hmrc.gov.uk
National Advice Line 0845 010 9000

RNLI SEA Check
www.rnli.org.uk/seacheck
0800 328 0600

British Waterways
www.boatsafetyscheme.com
01923 226422 or
0141 332 6939 in Scotland.

Conference of Yacht Cruising Clubs (CYCC)
www.cycc.org.uk

Health Advice when Travelling
(Department of Health)
www.doh.gov.uk/traveladvice

Radio Licensing Centre
PO Box 1495, Bristol BS99 3QS
www.radiolicencecentre.co.uk
0870 243 4433 (T)
0117 975 8911 (F)

The EPIRB Registry
MRCC Falmouth
Pendennis Point, Castle Drive
Falmouth, Cornwall TR11 4WZ
Email: epirb@mcga.gov.uk
www.mcga.gov.uk/flag/forms
01326 211569 (T)
01326 319264 (F)

Notice to Mariners:
www.nmwebsearch.com

Publications (Admiralty Chart Agent)
Sea Chest Nautical Bookshop
Queen Anne's Battery Marina
Plymouth, Devon PL4 0LP
Email: info@seachest.co.uk
01752 222012 (T)
01752 252679 (F)

Pet Travel Scheme
www.defra.gov.uk/animals/quarantine/index.htm
0870 241 1710
Email: infoline@mcga.gov.uk

Register of Shipping & Seamen
029 2044 8800
rss@mcga.gov.uk
www.mcga.gov.uk

INDEX

NOTES

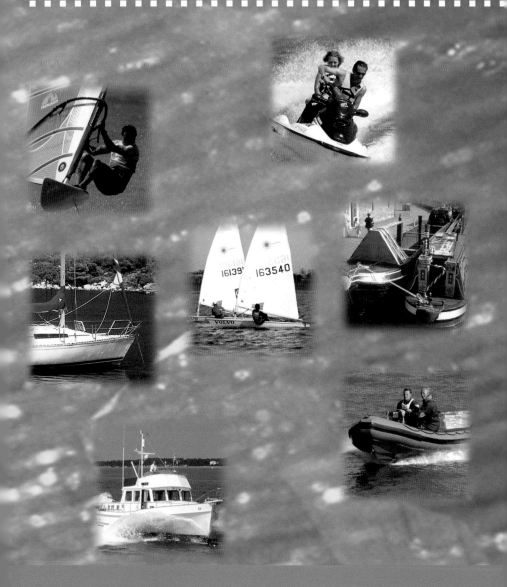

RYA *Membership*

Promoting and Protecting Boating
www.rya.org.uk

RYA Membership

Promoting and Protecting Boating

The RYA is the national organisation which represents the interests of everyone who goes boating for pleasure.

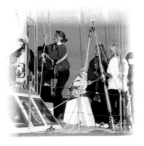

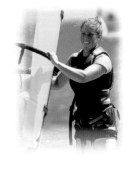

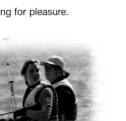

The greater the membership, the louder our voice when it comes to protecting members' interests.

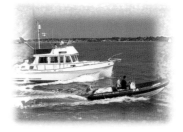

Apply for membership today, and support the RYA, to help the RYA support you.

Benefits of Membership

- Access to expert advice on all aspects of boating from legal wrangles to training matters
- Special members' discounts on a range of products and services including boat insurance, books, videos and class certificates
- Free issue of certificates of competence, increasingly asked for by everyone from overseas governments to holiday companies, insurance underwriters to boat hirers

- Access to the wide range of RYA publications, including the quarterly magazine
- Third Party insurance for windsurfing members
- Free Internet access with RYA-Online
- Special discounts on AA membership
- Regular offers in RYA Magazine
- ...and much more

Join now - membership form opposite

Join online at *www.rya.org.uk*

Visit our website for information, advice, members' services and web shop.

1 Important To help us comply with Data Protection legislation, please tick *either* Box A or Box B (you must tick Box A to ensure you receive the full benefits of RYA membership). The RYA will not pass your data to third parties.

☐ **A.** I wish to join the RYA and receive future information on member services, benefits (as listed in RYA Magazine and website) and offers.

☐ **B.** I wish to join the RYA but do not wish to receive future information on member services, benefits (as listed in RYA Magazine and website) and offers.

When completed, please send this form to: RYA, RYA House, Ensign Way, Hamble, Southampton, SO31 4YA

2

Title	Forename	Surname	Date of Birth		Male	Female
			D D / M M / Y Y		☐	☐
1.						
2.			D D / M M / Y Y		☐	☐
3.			D D / M M / Y Y		☐	☐
4.			D D / M M / Y Y		☐	☐

Address

Town   County   Post Code

Evening Telephone   Daytime Telephone

email

Signature: _____   Date: _____

3 Type of membership required: *(Tick Box)*

☐ **Personal** *Before 1 October 2005 annual rate £33 or £30 by Direct Debit*
                From 1 October 2005 annual rate £37 or £34 by Direct Debit

☐ **Under 21** *Before 1 October 2005 annual rate £11 (no reduction for Direct Debit)*
               From 1 October 2005 annual rate £12 (no reduction for Direct Debit)

☐ **Family*** *Before 1 October 2005 annual rate £50 or £47 by Direct Debit*
              From 1 October 2005 annual rate £56 or £52 by Direct Debit

* *Family Membership: 2 adults plus any under 21s all living at the same address*

4 Please tick ONE box to show your main boating interest.

☐ Yacht Racing   ☐ Yacht Cruising
☐ Dinghy Racing   ☐ Dinghy Cruising
☐ Personal Watercraft   ☐ Inland Waterways
☐ Powerboat Racing   ☐ Windsurfing
☐ Motor Boating   ☐ Sportsboats and RIBs

Please see Direct Debit form overleaf

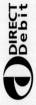

Instructions to your Bank or Building Society to pay by Direct Debit

Please complete this form and return it to:
Royal Yachting Association, RYA House, Ensign Way, Hamble, Southampton, Hampshire SO31 4YA

DIRECT Debit

To The Manager: _____ Bank/Building Society

Address: _____

Post Code: _____

2. Name(s) of account holder(s)

_____

3. Branch Sort Code

	—		—	

4. Bank or Building Society account number

Banks and Building Societies may not accept Direct Debit instructions for some types of account

Cash, Cheque, Postal Order enclosed £ _____
Made payable to the Royal Yachting Association

Office use only: Membership Number Allocated _____

077

Originators Identification Number

9	5	5	2	1	3

5. RYA Membership Number (For office use only)

_____

6. Instruction to pay your Bank or Building Society

Please pay Royal Yachting Association Direct Debits from the account detailed in this instruction subject to the safeguards assured by The Direct Debit Guarantee.
I understand that this instruction may remain with the Royal Yachting Association and, if so, details will be passed electronically to my Bank/Building Society.

Signature(s) _____

Date _____

Office use / Centre Stamp